OVERVIEW MAP KEY

EAST BAY

01. Wildcat Canyon Regional Park: Havey Canyon to Belgum Trail Loop 14
02. Redwood Regional Park: Big Loop Plus Graham and Dunn 19
03. Lake Chabot Regional Park: Lake Chabot Bicycle Loop 24
04. Briones Regional Park: Mott Peak Loop 29
05. Las Trampas Regional Park: Del Amigo Drop 34
06. Joseph D. Grant Ranch County Park: East Loops with Antler Point 39
07. Diablo Foothills: Foothills to Alamo Loop 44
08. Mission Peak: Mission Peak Loop 49
09. Mount Diablo State Park: Eagle Peak Loop 54
10. Black Diamond Mines Regional Preserve: Lark Trail to the Wall 59
11. Morgan Territory Regional Preserve: Big Southwest Loop 64
12. Morgan Territory Regional Preserve: Volvon Loop Variations 69

NORTH BAY

13. Marin Headlands: Big Southeast Loop with Coastal Trail 76
14. Marin Headlands: Northwest Loop from Tennessee Valley 81
15. Mount Tamalpais State Park: Hoo-Koo-E-Koo and Old Railroad Grade Loop 86
16. Mount Tamalpais State Park: Northern Loop—Rock Spring Road to Eldridge Grade via Bon Tempe Lake 91
17. China Camp State Park: Shoreline Trail and Oak Ridge Loop 96
18. Bolinas Ridge Trail: Bolinas Ridge Out-and-Back 101
19. Sleepy Hollow: Sleepy Hollow Out-and-Back 106
20. Helen Putnam Regional Park: "Don't Stop 'Til You Get Enough" 111

21. Rockville Hills Regional Park: The Black Map 116
22. Skyline Wilderness Park: Singlespeeder's Delight 121
23. Annadel State Park: Canyon Trail and Rough Go Loop 126
24. Annadel State Park: Warren Richardson—North Burma Loop 131
25. Shiloh Ranch Regional Park: Creekside Trail and Big Leaf Loop 137

SAN FRANCISCO

26. Mount Davidson: The Jungle at the Top of San Francisco 144
27. Mount Sutro: Mount Sutro Out-and-Back 149

SOUTH BAY

28. Pacifica: Sweeney Ridge Loop 156
29. Purisima Creek Redwoods: Whittemore Wonderland 161
30. Purisima Creek Redwoods: Grabtown Gulch Loop 166
31. El Corte de Madera Creek Open Space Preserve: Shoots and Ladders 171
32. El Corte de Madera Creek Open Space Preserve: Bear Gulch Loop 176
33. Pearson Arastradero Preserve: Acorn Trail Loop 181
34. Windy Hill Open Space Preserve: Windy Hill Out-and-Back 186
35. Coal Creek Open Space Preserve: Dog Bone Loop 191
36. Russian Ridge Open Space Preserve: Ancient Oaks Trail to Hawk Trail Loop 196
37. South Skyline Region Open Space Preserve: Four Parks Loop 201
38. Long Ridge Open Space Preserve: The Full Pond Loop 206
39. Almaden Quicksilver County Park: Mine Hill and Randol Trails Loop 211
40. Big Basin Redwoods State Park: Middle Ridge and Gazos Creek Loop 216

MOUNTAIN BIKE

SAN FRANCISCO BAY AREA

SKYE KRAFT

TO MOM—MY GUIDING SPIRIT AND THE MOST BEAUTIFUL PERSON I KNOW.

DISCLAIMER

This book is meant only as a guide to select trails within the San Francisco Bay Area and does not guarantee rider safety in any way—have fun, but you ride at your own risk. Neither Menasha Ridge Press nor Skye Kraft are liable for property loss or damage, personal injury, or death that result in any way from accessing or riding the trails described on the following pages. Be especially cautious when riding on or near boulders, steep inclines, and drop-offs, and do not attempt to explore terrain that may be beyond your abilities. To help ensure an uneventful ride, please read carefully the introduction to this book. Familiarize yourself thoroughly with the areas you intend to visit before venturing out. Ask questions and prepare for the unforeseen. Familiarize yourself with current weather reports, maps of the area you intend to visit, and any applicable trail regulations.

Library of Congress Cataloging-in-Publication Data:

Kraft, Skye.
Mountain bike! San Francisco Bay area : a wide-grin ride guide /
by Skye Kraft. — 1st ed.
p. cm.
ISBN-13: 978-0-89732-659-9
ISBN-10: 0-89732-659-8
1. Bicycle touring—California—San Francisco Bay Area—Guidebooks.
2. San Francisco Bay Area (Calif.)—Guidebooks. I. Title.
GV1045.5.C22S2654 2008
796.6309794'6—dc22
2008010731

MENASHA RIDGE PRESS
P.O. BOX 43673
BIRMINGHAM, ALABAMA 35243
WWW.MENASHARIDGE.COM

CONTENTS

ACKNOWLEDGMENTS   vii

ABOUT THE AUTHOR   ix

PREFACE   x

RECOMMENDED RIDES   xiii

INTRODUCTION   1

EAST BAY   13

01 Wildcat Canyon Regional Park: Havey Canyon to Belgum Trail Loop 14

02 Redwood Regional Park: Big Loop Plus Graham and Dunn............................ 19

03 Lake Chabot Regional Park: Lake Chabot Bicycle Loop 24

04 Briones Regional Park: Mott Peak Loop 29

05 Las Trampas Regional Park: Del Amigo Drop 34

06 Joseph D. Grant Ranch County Park: East Loops with Antler Point 39

07 Diablo Foothills: Foothills to Alamo Loop 44

08 Mission Peak: Mission Peak Loop 49

09 Mount Diablo State Park: Eagle Peak Loop... 54

10 Black Diamond Mines Regional Preserve: Lark Trail to the Wall 59

11 Morgan Territory Regional Preserve: Big Southwest Loop 64

12 Morgan Territory Regional Preserve: Volvon Loop Variations 69

NORTH BAY   75

13 Marin Headlands: Big Southeast Loop with Coastal Trail 76

14 Marin Headlands: Northwest Loop from Tennessee Valley........................... 81

15 Mount Tamalpais State Park: Hoo-Koo-E-Koo and
Railroad Grade Loop 86

16 Mount Tamalpais State Park: Northern Loop—Rock Spring Road to
Eldridge Grade via Bon Tempe Lake 91

17 China Camp State Park: Shoreline Trail and Oak Ridge Loop 96

18 Bolinas Ridge Trail: Bolinas Ridge Out-and-Back................................ 101

19 Sleepy Hollow: Sleepy Hollow Out-and-Back 106

20 Helen Putnam Regional Park: "Don't Stop 'Til You Get Enough" 111

21 Rockville Hills Regional Park: The Black Map 116

22 Skyline Wilderness Park: Singlespeeder's Delight 121

23 Annadel State Park: Canyon Trail and Rough Go Loop 126

Contents

24 Annadel State Park: Warren Richardson–North Burma Loop 131

25 Shiloh Ranch Regional Park: Creekside Trail and Big Leaf Loop 137

SAN FRANCISCO   143

26 Mount Davidson: The Jungle at the Top of San Francisco 144

27 Mount Sutro: Mount Sutro Out-and-Back 149

SOUTH BAY   155

28 Pacifica: Sweeney Ridge Loop..156

29 Purisima Creek Redwoods: Whittemore Wonderland....................................161

30 Purisima Creek Redwoods: Grabtown Gulch Loop 166

31 El Corte de Madera Creek Open Space Preserve: Shoots and Ladders 171

32 El Corte de Madera Creek Open Space Preserve: Bear Gulch Loop................176

33 Pearson Arastradero Preserve: Acorn Trail Loop 181

34 Windy Hill Open Space Preserve: Windy Hill Out-and-Back 186

35 Coal Creek Open Space Preserve: Dog Bone Loop...............................191

36 Russian Ridge Open Space Preserve: Ancient Oaks Trail
   to Hawk Trail Loop 196

37 South Skyline Region Open Space Preserve: Four Parks Loop...................... 201

38 Long Ridge Open Space Preserve: The Full Pond Loop 206

39 Almaden Quicksilver County Park: Mine Hill and Randol Trails Loop 211

40 Big Basin Redwoods State Park: Middle Ridge and Gazos Creek Loop...........216

APPENDIXES

Appendix A: Bicycling Clubs in the Greater San Francisco Bay Area....................224

Appendix B: Bicycling Retailers in the Greater San Francisco Bay Area...............226

INDEX   234

ACKNOWLEDGMENTS

This book is the realization of a life-long dream of mine—to become an author—and I would like to express my immense gratitude to Menasha Ridge Press for selecting me for this unbelievable project. From my parents, who raised me in a beautiful rural environment and helped me purchase my first mountain bike, to all the people I've met on my various cycling adventures—there are so many who have helped push me to this point in my life. Jared and Jason: thanks for being the two other musketeers on all of our teenage mountain biking adventures; and thanks to Big Jim for being the pilot and playing the Creedence. Thanks to Yuri Hauswald for asking me to ride on one of the first Mudpuppy teams back in the day. Thanks to Roald Dahl, Richard Speakes, all of my UCLA literature professors, and all of the authors I've loved in my life for the continued inspiration to write and the guiding of my voice. Many thanks go out to everyone from the various parks systems I visited who answered my questions, big and small. Special thanks to my friend William Arenander, baron of the Sonoma County Regional Parks system and connoisseur of the hiking trails of the world, for advising me on both the functional and political intricacies of the Northern California parks systems. I want to express my appreciation to the San Francisco Bicycle Coalition for being a much needed human-powered advocate in the Bay Area. Love to all my coworkers at Linden Lab for understanding why I could never come out and play after work. Aubrey, thanks for just being my sister and for pioneering our life in the city. And last but not least—thank you, Justine, for putting up with me during one very busy year.

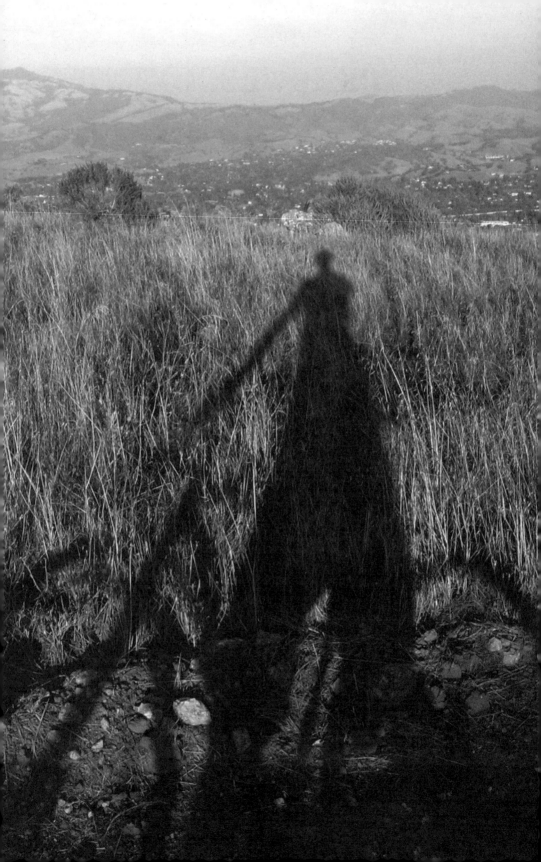

ABOUT THE AUTHOR

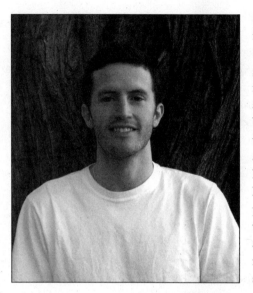

Skye Kraft is a native of the Bay Area, having grown up on 40 acres in eastern Santa Rosa, in the hills below Hood Mountain Regional Park. Due to the rough, hilly 12-mile road into town (4 of those miles were dirt), at age 12 Skye took up mountain biking to be able to visit friends, and started logging the miles. He began racing mountain bikes at age 13 and switched to road racing in college. He took that as far as the semi-pro level, scoring a handful of strong results in pro-level events before drifting away from the race scene in 2006. Skye remains an avid cyclist and advocate for bicycle commuting. Contact Skye for book updates at skyekraft@skyekraft.com.

PREFACE

I fell in love with bikes because they were fun: challenging your friend as to who could ride their BMX bike in the tightest circle, for the longest time, without falling down is just the kind of stupid physics that any great childhood is built on. I became addicted to cycling out of necessity: simply needing a way to get from point A to point B and back before I was old enough to drive a car. I grew up in the country, seven miles from town—over the hills, far away, down a long and winding dirt road—and before I got my driver's license, in order to see my town-bound friends I either had to beg my parents for a ride or get over that hill under my own power. Being the self-sufficient personality that I am, I chose the latter. Rather than walk, run, or hitchhike everywhere, I opted for the much more efficient and fun (sorry, runners) mountain bike. It was an eye-opening experience for my teenage self, to go from feeling almost completely isolated to completely connected, and trading only a couple of sore legs for the effort.

It didn't take long for my friends and myself to get into mountain bike racing, and we raced all over Northern California, thanks to our parents' chaperoning. That was when I got my first taste of many of the rides presented in this book. We raced under the mantles of Tinker Juarez, John Tomac, and Julie Furtado in the glorious young days of the sport, which rose rapidly to Olympic prominence. During college I switched to racing road bikes, based in large part on the Lance Armstrong influence. I spent the first couple years out of college pursuing the professional road-racing circuit, and though I did get close, the arc of my success fell just short of the pressures-of-life wall, so I swapped my skinny-tired race bike for a single-speed 29er mountain bike commuter and an office career and re-sparked my love of the trails.

Now I live and work in San Francisco, and I choose the bike as my primary form of transportation—I wouldn't have it any other way. Yes, I do own a car, and I do respect the public transportation system here, but the bottom line is that San Francisco is a rider's city and the Bay Area is a rider's region. Whether you are a commuter, road cyclist, or mountain biker, this region is one of the most amazing places to pedal a bicycle, and the 40 rides described in this book represent the best and most accessible legal mountain bike trails to be experienced within a 70-mile radius of the San Francisco city center. Some of these rides I grew up with, some now serve as my de facto gym membership (that is, close enough to get to after work), and many I experienced for the first time while researching this book.

Annadel State Park in Santa Rosa was the stomping ground for me and my friends when we were growing up. From Upper Steve's Trail to the Lake Ilsanjo Trail, that park still holds rein over my mountain biking heart. There are some mythical aspects of my mountain biking youth, such as descending what is now Fountain Grove Parkway in Santa Rosa when it was still just a massive dirt cut through the chaparral mountain; the old Ring of Fire races put on by Gianni Cyclery out in Occidental; and the triple black diamond Waterfall Trail in Annadel—all things that no longer exist except in memories, a few medals, and a couple of scars. The very nature of mountain biking, and outdoors activities in general, in Northern California has an almost transient value. Every day, it seems, we lose one more trail to anti-biker political movement, or one more open-space area to housing development.

It was incredible to discover parks that had previously escaped my notice, such as El Corte de Madera, Morgan Territory, and Purisima Creek. Working on this book also gave me perfect reason to revisit Skyline Wilderness Park, in Napa, site of the upcoming 2008 Singlespeed World Championships (SSWC). I had raced in Skyline Wilderness Park a number of times as a teenager, but when I revisited it for purposes of this book, I was blown away by the quality of trails and unrivaled access for mountain bikers. Any one of the above parks poses as a rival to Annadel for the affections of my heart, but in the end Annadel is like family to me, and only extreme trail closure could break that bond.

No matter what kind of riding you're looking for, the Bay Area has it, with the exception of shuttled downhillers' runs—for those you'll have to wait until summer, trek up to Tahoe, and make use of the off-season ski parks. What I have sought to provide in this book is the best rides in the best parks, all within a 60-mile radius of San Francisco (except for Big Basin, which is 70 miles from the city). If you're a city dweller, like myself, then each of these rides makes an excellent day trip. Wherever possible I have sought to create a loop. I have usually opted for a medium-to-large-sized loop and offered advice on the best ways to shorten or lengthen a ride to taste. I am personally a singletrack fiend and have focused my rides around that elixir of trail construction. Fortunately for you fire-road lovers, the restrictive access rights in many parks prevent bikes from touching the singletracks, and this has created a great blend of trail types—otherwise my intention would be to fill this book with the skinny trail.

Where it was convenient, I included "no car necessary" directions for getting to these parks from San Francisco. This isn't to say that one wouldn't be able to arrange public transportation to most of the rides in this book, but considering space constraints and the need to provide car-centric directions, I had to omit excessively complicated directions, such as those that required five bus transfers and a comic's sense of timing. East Bay and South Bay are the winners in terms of ease of public transportation, for they are blessed with the BART train, whose egress to the north the city of Marin has inconveniently prevented, thereby restricting sensible commuters north of the Golden Gate Bridge to the less efficient bus option. However, unlike the Bay Bridge to the East Bay, bikes are allowed to ride across the Golden Gate, and one of my favorite evening rides is to jet across the bridge and around one of the loops in the Marin Headlands, or maybe even up to China Camp if I've got a little extra time.

When cycling across the Golden Gate Bridge, make every effort to ride on the west side of the bridge. This side is open only during specific hours of the day, and these hours change slightly with each season, but try to ride on that side first. If you try to ride along the east side of the bridge during peak tourist hours, let's just say that you will be very frustrated. Here are some more tips for riding in San Francisco:

- First, go to one of these two places: **http://bicycling.511.org/maps.htm or www.sfbike.org/download/map.pdf** and download the comprehensive San Francisco bike map.
- Second, *do not ride on any street with more than four lanes.* There are enough bike routes lacing the city that it is unnecessary to endanger yourself and impede the drivers on roads such as Van Ness Avenue, Geary Boulevard, Oak Street, or 19th Avenue, to name just a few. If you find yourself on one of these roads, check one street to the right or left, for there is almost always a smaller, bike-friendly street running parallel to these mini-highways. Just look for the little green signs with a bike and a number—those indicate bike routes.
- Third, don't expect that you are completely safe from cars in Golden Gate Park, except on weekends, when it is closed to vehicles. Just as there are wayward cyclists trying to ride the big streets, there are also wayward drivers who feel it is necessary to commute through the park as though *it* were a highway.

The above tips will be helpful should you decide to string together all of the off-road riding in the city (Golden Gate Park, Mount Davidson, Mount Sutro, Glen Canyon, John McLaren), or if you just plan to explore the city by bike. If I had a magic wand and a time machine, I would reshape this city with a far-reaching, pan-directional BART; efficient north–south autoroutes tunneled *beneath* Golden Gate Park; foot and bicycle regulations through Broadway Tunnel; and bike lanes on the Bay Bridge. Unfortunately, I don't have either of those, so things will have to stay as they are.

If you need to get away from the pavement altogether and get up to a tall place with a view, then you'll want to climb up some of the taller peaks in the area, like Mount Diablo, Mount Tamalpais, or Mission Peak. Despite all of the development that's happened in the last 20 years, there's still a lot of dirt, trees, and rocks to love in the San Francisco Bay Area, and there's no better way to do it than on a mountain bike. Live. Bike.

RECOMMENDED RIDES

Rides 1–5 Miles

07 Diablo Foothills: Foothills to Alamo Loop 44

14 Marin Headlands: Northwest Loop from Tennessee Valley 81

20 Helen Putnam Regional Park: "Don't Stop 'Til You Get Enough" 111

25 Shiloh Ranch Regional Park: Creekside Trail and Big Leaf Loop 137

26 Mount Davidson: The Jungle at the Top of San Francisco 144

27 Mount Sutro: Mount Sutro Out-and-Back 149

30 Purisima Creek Redwoods: Grabtown Gulch Loop 166

33 Pearson Arastradero Preserve: Acorn Trail Loop 181

34 Windy Hill Open Space Preserve: Windy Hill Out-and-Back 186

35 Coal Creek Open Space Preserve: Dog Bone Loop 191

36 Russian Ridge Open Space Preserve: Ancient Oaks Trail to Hawk Trail Loop 196

Rides 6–10 Miles

02 Redwood Regional Park: Big Loop Plus Graham and Dunn 19

04 Briones Regional Park: Mott Peak Loop 29

05 Las Trampas Regional Park: Del Amigo Drop 34

08 Mission Peak: Mission Peak Loop 49

09 Mount Diablo State Park: Eagle Peak Loop 54

10 Black Diamond Mines Regional Preserve: Lark Trail to the Wall 59

12 Morgan Territory Regional Preserve: Volvon Loop Variations 69

13 Marin Headlands: Big Southeast Loop with Coastal Trail 76

15 Mount Tamalpais State Park: Hoo-Koo-E-Koo and Old Railroad Grade Loop 86

17 China Camp State Park: Shoreline Trail and Oak Ridge Loop 96

19 Sleepy Hollow: Sleepy Hollow Out-and-Back 106

21 Rockville Hills Regional Park: The Black Map 116

22 Skyline Wilderness Park: Singlespeeder's Delight 121

23 Annadel State Park: Canyon Trail and Rough Go Loop 126

28 Pacifica: Sweeney Ridge Loop 156

29 Purisima Creek Redwoods: Whittemore Wonderland 161

31 El Corte de Madera Creek Open Space Preserve: Shoots and Ladders 171

32 El Corte de Madera Creek Open Space Preserve: Bear Gulch Loop 176

37 South Skyline Region Open Space Preserve: Four Parks Loop 201

38 Long Ridge Open Space Preserve: The Full Pond Loop 206

Rides 11–20 Miles

01 Wildcat Canyon Regional Park: Havey Canyon to Belgum Trail Loop 14

03 Lake Chabot Regional Park: Lake Chabot Bicycle Loop 24

06 Joseph D. Grant Ranch County Park: East Loops with Antler Point 39

11 Morgan Territory Regional Preserve: Big Southwest Loop 64

16 Mount Tamalpais State Park: Northern Loop—Rock Spring Road to Eldridge Grade via Bon Tempe Lake 91

24 Annadel State Park: Warren
Richardson–North Burma Loop 131

39 Almaden Quicksilver County Park: Mine
Hill and Randol Trails Loop 211

40 Big Basin Redwoods State Park: Middle
Ridge and Gazos Creek Loop 216

Rides More than 20 Miles

18 Bolinas Ridge Trail: Bolinas
Ridge Out-and-Back 101

Rides with 0 to 1,000 Feet of Climbing

20 Helen Putnam Regional Park: "Don't Stop
'Til You Get Enough" 111

23 Annadel State Park: Canyon Trail and
Rough Go Loop 126

25 Shiloh Ranch Regional Park: Creekside
Trail and Big Leaf Loop 137

26 Mount Davidson: The Jungle at the Top of
San Francisco 144

27 Mount Sutro: Mount Sutro
Out-and-Back 149

33 Pearson Arastradero Preserve: Acorn Trail
Loop 181

Rides with 1,001 to 2,000 Feet of Climbing

04 Briones Regional Park: Mott Peak
Loop 29

07 Diablo Foothills: Foothills to Alamo
Loop 44

12 Morgan Territory Regional Preserve:
Volvon Loop Variations 69

14 Marin Headlands: Northwest Loop from
Tennessee Valley 81

15 Mount Tamalpais State Park: Hoo-Koo-E-
Koo and Old Railroad Grade Loop 86

17 China Camp State Park: Shoreline Trail and
Oak Ridge Loop 96

21 Rockville Hills Regional Park:
The Black Map 116

28 Pacifica: Sweeney Ridge Loop 156

34 Windy Hill Open Space Preserve:
Windy Hill Out-and-Back 186

35 Coal Creek Open Space Preserve: Dog
Bone Loop 191

36 Russian Ridge Open Space Preserve:
Ancient Oaks Trail to Hawk Trail
Loop 196

38 Long Ridge Open Space Preserve:
The Full Pond Loop 206

Rides with 2,001 to 3,000 Feet of Climbing

01 Wildcat Canyon Regional Park: Havey
Canyon to Belgum Trail Loop 14

02 Redwood Regional Park: Big Loop Plus
Graham and Dunn 19

03 Lake Chabot Regional Park: Lake Chabot
Bicycle Loop 24

05 Las Trampas Regional Park: Del Amigo
Drop 34

06 Joseph D. Grant Ranch County Park: East
Loops with Antler Point 39

08 Mission Peak: Mission Peak Loop 49

09 Mount Diablo State Park: Eagle Peak
Loop 54

10 Black Diamond Mines Regional Preserve:
Lark Trail to the Wall 59

13 Marin Headlands: Big Southeast Loop with
Coastal Trail 76

19 Sleepy Hollow: Sleepy Hollow
Out-and-Back 106

22 Skyline Wilderness Park: Singlespeeder's
Delight 121

24 Annadel State Park: Warren Richardson–
North Burma Loop 131

29 Purisima Creek Redwoods: Whittemore
Wonderland 161

30 Purisima Creek Redwoods: Grabtown
Gulch Loop 166

31 El Corte de Madera Creek Open Space
Preserve: Shoots and Ladders 171

32 El Corte de Madera Creek Open Space
Preserve: Bear Gulch Loop 176

37 South Skyline Region Open Space
Preserve: Four Parks Loop 201

39 Almaden Quicksilver County Park: Mine
Hill and Randol Trails Loop 211

Rides with More than 3,000 Feet of Climbing

11 Morgan Territory Regional Preserve: Big Southwest Loop   64

16 Mount Tamalpais State Park: Northern Loop—Rock Spring Road to Eldridge Grade via Bon Tempe Lake   91

18 Bolinas Ridge Trail: Bolinas Ridge Out-and-Back   101

40 Big Basin Redwoods State Park: Middle Ridge and Gazos Creek Loop   216

Rides with Jumps

03 Lake Chabot Regional Park: Lake Chabot Bicycle Loop   24

10 Black Diamond Mines Regional Preserve: Lark Trail to the Wall   59

23 Annadel State Park: Canyon Trail and Rough Go Loop   126

31 El Corte de Madera Creek Open Space Preserve: Shoots and Ladders   171

32 El Corte de Madera Creek Open Space Preserve: Bear Gulch Loop   176

40 Big Basin Redwoods State Park: Middle Ridge and Gazos Creek Loop   216

Rides with Extreme Drops

01 Wildcat Canyon Regional Park: Havey Canyon to Belgum Trail Loop   14

05 Las Trampas Regional Park: Del Amigo Drop   34

09 Mount Diablo State Park: Eagle Peak Loop   54

15 Mount Tamalpais State Park: Hoo-Koo-E-Koo and Old Railroad Grade Loop   86

17 China Camp State Park: Shoreline Trail and Oak Ridge Loop   96

21 Rockville Hills Regional Park: The Black Map   116

22 Skyline Wilderness Park: Singlespeeder's Delight   121

23 Annadel State Park: Canyon Trail and Rough Go Loop   126

24 Annadel State Park: Warren Richardson–North Burma Loop   131

29 Purisima Creek Redwoods: Whittemore Wonderland   161

31 El Corte de Madera Creek Open Space Preserve: Shoots and Ladders   171

32 El Corte de Madera Creek Open Space Preserve: Bear Gulch Loop   176

37 South Skyline Region Open Space Preserve: Four Parks Loop   201

Lonely Rides

03 Lake Chabot Regional Park: Lake Chabot Bicycle Loop   24

04 Briones Regional Park: Mott Peak Loop   29

06 Joseph D. Grant Ranch County Park: East Loops with Antler Point   39

09 Mount Diablo State Park: Eagle Peak Loop   54

10 Black Diamond Mines Regional Preserve: Lark Trail to the Wall   59

11 Morgan Territory Regional Preserve: Big Southwest Loop   64

18 Bolinas Ridge Trail: Bolinas Ridge Out-and-Back   101

29 Purisima Creek Redwoods: Whittemore Wonderland   161

36 Russian Ridge Open Space Preserve: Ancient Oaks Trail to Hawk Trail Loop   196

37 South Skyline Region Open Space Preserve: Four Parks Loop   201

38 Long Ridge Open Space Preserve: The Full Pond Loop   206

40 Big Basin Redwoods State Park: Middle Ridge and Gazos Creek Loop   216

Crowded Rides

01 Wildcat Canyon Regional Park: Havey Canyon to Belgum Trail Loop   14

02 Redwood Regional Park: Big Loop Plus Graham and Dunn   19

07 Diablo Foothills: Foothills to Alamo Loop   44

15 Mount Tamalpais State Park: Hoo-Koo-E-Koo and Old Railroad Grade Loop   86

16 Mount Tamalpais State Park: Northern Loop—Rock Spring Road to Eldridge Grade via Bon Tempe Lake 91

17 China Camp State Park: Shoreline Trail and Oak Ridge Loop 96

21 Rockville Hills Regional Park: The Black Map 116

31 El Corte de Madera Creek Open Space Preserve: Shoots and Ladders 171

32 El Corte de Madera Creek Open Space Preserve: Bear Gulch Loop 176

33 Pearson Arastradero Preserve: Acorn Trail Loop 181

Best-maintained Rides

02 Redwood Regional Park: Big Loop Plus Graham and Dunn 19

10 Black Diamond Mines Regional Preserve: Lark Trail to the Wall 59

12 Morgan Territory Regional Preserve: Volvon Loop Variations 69

13 Marin Headlands: Big Southeast Loop with Coastal Trail 76

14 Marin Headlands: Northwest Loop from Tennessee Valley 81

20 Helen Putnam Regional Park: "Don't Stop 'Til You Get Enough" 111

21 Rockville Hills Regional Park: The Black Map 116

22 Skyline Wilderness Park: Singlespeeder's Delight 121

23 Annadel State Park: Canyon Trail and Rough Go Loop 126

24 Annadel State Park: Warren Richardson–North Burma Loop 131

29 Purisima Creek Redwoods: Whittemore Wonderland 161

31 El Corte de Madera Creek Open Space Preserve: Shoots and Ladders 171

32 El Corte de Madera Creek Open Space Preserve: Bear Gulch Loop 176

36 Russian Ridge Open Space Preserve: Ancient Oaks Trail to Hawk Trail Loop 196

Easy Rides

03 Lake Chabot Regional Park: Lake Chabot Bicycle Loop 24

14 Marin Headlands: Northwest Loop from Tennessee Valley 81

15 Mount Tamalpais State Park: Hoo-Koo-E-Koo and Old Railroad Grade Loop 86

20 Helen Putnam Regional Park: "Don't Stop 'Til You Get Enough" 111

21 Rockville Hills Regional Park: The Black Map 116

25 Shiloh Ranch Regional Park: Creekside Trail and Big Leaf Loop 137

33 Pearson Arastradero Preserve: Acorn Trail Loop 181

36 Russian Ridge Open Space Preserve: Ancient Oaks Trail to Hawk Trail Loop 196

Flat Rides

20 Helen Putnam Regional Park: "Don't Stop 'Til You Get Enough" 111

33 Pearson Arastradero Preserve: Acorn Trail Loop 181

Steep Rides

01 Wildcat Canyon Regional Park: Havey Canyon to Belgum Trail Loop 14

02 Redwood Regional Park: Big Loop Plus Graham and Dunn 19

03 Lake Chabot Regional Park: Lake Chabot Bicycle Loop 24

04 Briones Regional Park: Mott Peak Loop 29

05 Las Trampas Regional Park: Del Amigo Drop 34

06 Joseph D. Grant Ranch County Park: East Loops with Antler Point 39

07 Diablo Foothills: Foothills to Alamo Loop 44

08 Mission Peak: Mission Peak Loop 49

09 Mount Diablo State Park: Eagle Peak Loop 54

10 Black Diamond Mines Regional Preserve: Lark Trail to the Wall 59

11 Morgan Territory Regional Preserve: Big Southwest Loop 64

12 Morgan Territory Regional Preserve: Volvon Loop Variations 69

13 Marin Headlands: Big Southeast Loop with Coastal Trail 76

19 Sleepy Hollow: Sleepy Hollow Out-and-Back 106

28 Pacifica: Sweeney Ridge Loop 156

29 Purisima Creek Redwoods: Whittemore Wonderland 161

30 Purisima Creek Redwoods: Grabtown Gulch Loop 166

34 Windy Hill Open Space Preserve: Windy Hill Out-and-Back 186

40 Big Basin Redwoods State Park: Middle Ridge and Gazos Creek Loop 216

Scenic Rides

01–40: All 14–216

05 Las Trampas Regional Park: Del Amigo Drop 34

11 Morgan Territory Regional Preserve: Big Southwest Loop 64

12 Morgan Territory Regional Preserve: Volvon Loop Variations 69

13 Marin Headlands: Big Southeast Loop with Coastal Trail 76

14 Marin Headlands: Northwest Loop from Tennessee Valley 81

16 Mount Tamalpais State Park: Northern Loop—Rock Spring Road to Eldridge Grade via Bon Tempe Lake 91

17 China Camp State Park: Shoreline Trail and Oak Ridge Loop 96

18 Bolinas Ridge Trail: Bolinas Ridge Out-and-Back 101

29 Purisima Creek Redwoods: Whittemore Wonderland 161

30 Purisima Creek Redwoods: Grabtown Gulch Loop 166

38 Long Ridge Open Space Preserve: The Full Pond Loop 206

40 Big Basin Redwoods State Park: Middle Ridge and Gazos Creek Loop 216

Urban Rides

26 Mount Davidson: The Jungle at the Top of San Francisco 144

27 Mount Sutro: Mount Sutro Out-and-Back 149

Creek and River Rides

01 Wildcat Canyon Regional Park: Havey Canyon to Belgum Trail Loop 14

09 Mount Diablo State Park: Eagle Peak Loop 54

11 Morgan Territory Regional Preserve: Big Southwest Loop 64

12 Morgan Territory Regional Preserve: Volvon Loop Variations 69

16 Mount Tamalpais State Park: Northern Loop—Rock Spring Road to Eldridge Grade via Bon Tempe Lake 91

22 Skyline Wilderness Park: Singlespeeder's Delight 121

24 Annadel State Park: Warren Richardson–North Burma Loop 131

25 Shiloh Ranch Regional Park: Creekside Trail and Big Leaf Loop 137

29 Purisima Creek Redwoods: Whittemore Wonderland 161

30 Purisima Creek Redwoods: Grabtown Gulch Loop 166

31 El Corte de Madera Creek Open Space Preserve: Shoots and Ladders 171

32 El Corte de Madera Creek Open Space Preserve: Bear Gulch Loop 176

33 Pearson Arastradero Preserve: Acorn Trail Loop 181

37 South Skyline Region Open Space Preserve: Four Parks Loop 201

38 Long Ridge Open Space Preserve: The Full Pond Loop 206

40 Big Basin Redwoods State Park: Middle Ridge and Gazos Creek Loop 216

Lake Rides

03 Lake Chabot Regional Park: Lake Chabot Bicycle Loop 24

06 Joseph D. Grant Ranch County Park: East
   Loops with Antler Point   39

16 Mount Tamalpais State Park: Northern
   Loop—Rock Spring Road to Eldridge
   Grade via Bon Tempe Lake   91

17 China Camp State Park: Shoreline Trail and
   Oak Ridge Loop   96

21 Rockville Hills Regional Park: The Black
   Map   116

22 Skyline Wilderness Park: Singlespeeder's
   Delight   121

23 Annadel State Park: Canyon Trail and
   Rough Go Loop   126

24 Annadel State Park: Warren Richardson–
   North Burma Loop   131

37 South Skyline Region Open Space
   Preserve: Four Parks Loop   201

39 Almaden Quicksilver County Park: Mine
   Hill and Randol Trails Loop   211

Wildflower Rides

01 Wildcat Canyon Regional Park: Havey
   Canyon to Belgum Trail Loop   14

04 Briones Regional Park: Mott Peak
   Loop   29

06 Joseph D. Grant Ranch County Park: East
   Loops with Antler Point   39

09 Mount Diablo State Park: Eagle Peak
   Loop   54

11 Morgan Territory Regional Preserve: Big
   Southwest Loop   64

18 Bolinas Ridge Trail: Bolinas Ridge Out-
   and-Back   101

20 Helen Putnam Regional Park: "Don't Stop
   'Til You Get Enough"   111

23 Annadel State Park: Canyon Trail and
   Rough Go Loop   126

24 Annadel State Park: Warren Richardson–
   North Burma Loop   131

25 Shiloh Ranch Regional Park: Creekside
   Trail and Big Leaf Loop   137

29 Purisima Creek Redwoods: Whittemore
   Wonderland   161

33 Pearson Arastradero Preserve: Acorn Trail
   Loop   181

34 Windy Hill Open Space Preserve:
   Windy Hill Out-and-Back   186

36 Russian Ridge Open Space Preserve:
   Ancient Oaks Trail to Hawk Trail
   Loop   196

38 Long Ridge Open Space Preserve:
   The Full Pond Loop   206

Wildlife Rides

01 Wildcat Canyon Regional Park: Havey
   Canyon to Belgum Trail Loop   14

03 Lake Chabot Regional Park: Lake Chabot
   Bicycle Loop   24

04 Briones Regional Park: Mott Peak
   Loop   29

06 Joseph D. Grant Ranch County Park: East
   Loops with Antler Point   39

09 Mount Diablo State Park: Eagle Peak
   Loop   54

10 Black Diamond Mines Regional Preserve:
   Lark Trail to the Wall   59

11 Morgan Territory Regional Preserve: Big
   Southwest Loop   64

13 Marin Headlands: Big Southeast Loop with
   Coastal Trail   76

22 Skyline Wilderness Park: Singlespeeder's
   Delight   121

23 Annadel State Park: Canyon Trail and
   Rough Go Loop   126

24 Annadel State Park: Warren Richardson–
   North Burma Loop   131

36 Russian Ridge Open Space Preserve: Ancient Oaks Trail to Hawk Trail Loop   196

37 South Skyline Region Open Space Preserve: Four Parks Loop   201

40 Big Basin Redwoods State Park: Middle
   Ridge and Gazos Creek Loop   216

INTRODUCTION

How to Use This Guidebook

Select the type of ride you are looking for from the breakdown of ride categories, or just take a look at the overview map to see what kind of rides are available closest to you. Read the "Key At-a-Glance Information" and "In Brief" sections for your chosen rides; these will give you a better idea about what to expect in terms of ride difficulty, as well as what facilities are available at the trailhead. The ride descriptions give a detailed run-through of each ride, highlighting the more exciting aspects and clarifying some of the directions at the more confusing trail junctions.

The Overview Map and Overview-map Key

Use the overview map on the inside front cover to assess the location of each ride's primary trailhead. Each ride's number appears on the overview map, on the map key facing the overview map, in the table of contents, and at the top of the ride description's pages.

Trail Maps

Each ride contains a detailed map that shows the trailhead, the route, significant features, facilities, and topographic landmarks, such as creeks, overlooks, and peaks. The author gathered map data by carrying a GPS unit Garmin Etrex Legend while hiking. GPS data was downloaded into a digital mapping program DeLorme TOPO USA 7.0 and processed by expert cartographers to produce the highly accurate maps found in this book. Each trailhead's GPS coordinates are included with each profile (see below).

Elevation Profiles

Corresponding directly to the trail map, each ride contains a detailed elevation profile. The elevation profile provides a quick look at the trail from the side, enabling you to visualize how the trail rises and falls. Note the number of feet between each tick mark on the vertical axis (the height scale). To avoid making flat rides look steep and steep rides appear flat, appropriate height scales are used throughout the book to provide an accurate image of the ride's climbing difficulty. Elevation profiles for loop rides show total distance; those for out-and-back rides show only one-way distance.

GPS Trailhead Coordinates

In addition to GPS-based maps, this book includes the GPS coordinates for each trailhead in two formats: latitude–longitude and UTM (Universal Transverse Mercator). Latitude–longitude coordinates employ a grid system that indicates your location by crossroading a line that runs north to south with a line that runs east to west. Lines of latitude are parallel and run east to west. The 0° line of latitude is the equator. Lines of longitude are not parallel, run north to south, and converge at the North and South poles. The 0° line of longitude passes through Greenwich, England.

Topographic maps show latitude and longitude as well as UTM grid lines. Known as UTM coordinates, the numbers index a specific point, also using a grid method. The survey information, or datum, used to arrive at the coordinates in this book is WGS84 (versus NAD27 or WGS83). For readers who own a GPS unit, whether handheld or onboard a vehicle, the latitude–longitude or UTM coordinates provided on the first page of each ride may be entered into the GPS unit. Just make sure your GPS unit is set to navigate using WGS84 datum. Now you can navigate directly to the trailhead.

Trailheads in parking areas can be reached by car, but some rides still require a short walk or ride to reach the official trailhead from the parking area. In those cases, a handheld unit is necessary to continue the GPS navigation process. That said, readers can easily access all trailheads in this book without a GPS unit, by using the directions given, the overview map, and the trail map, which shows at least one significant road leading into the area. But for those who enjoy using the latest GPS technology to navigate, the necessary data has been provided. A brief explanation of the UTM coordinates for Mission Peak Loop (page 49) follows.

UTM Zone   10S
Easting   0596620
Northing   4151170

The UTM zone number 10 refers to one of the 60 vertical zones of the UTM projection, each of which is 6 degrees wide. The "S" refers to horizontal zones, each of which is 8 degrees wide except for Zone X (12 degrees wide). The easting number 0596620 indicates in meters how far east or west a point is from the central meridian of the zone. Increasing easting coordinates on a topographic map or on your GPS screen indicate that you are moving east; decreasing easting coordinates indicate that you are moving west. The northing number 4151170 references in meters how far you are from the equator. Increasing northing coordinates indicate you are traveling north; decreasing northing coordinates indicate you are traveling south. To learn more about how to enhance your outdoor experiences with GPS technology, refer to *GPS Outdoors: A Practical Guide for Outdoor Enthusiasts* (Menasha Ridge Press).

Ride Description

Each ride contains a detailed description of the route from beginning to end. The description is the heart of each ride. Here, the author provides a summary of the trail's essence and highlights any extras the ride has to offer. The route is clearly outlined, including landmarks, side trips, and possible alternate routes along the way. The main narrative is enhanced with an "In Brief" description of the ride, a Key at-a-Glance Information box, and driving directions to the trailhead. Many rides include a note on nearby activities, such as where to grab a cold brew after the ride.

In Brief

A "taste of the ride": think of this section as a snapshot focused on the historic landmarks, scenic vistas, and other sights you may encounter on the ride.

Key at-a-Glance Information

The information in the key at-a-glance boxes gives you quick statistics and specifics of each ride.

Length The length of the ride from start to finish (total distance traveled). There may be options to shorten or extend the ride, but the mileage corresponds to the described ride. Consult the ride description for help deciding on how to customize the ride for your ability or time constraints.

Configuration A description of what the ride might look like from overhead. Rides can be loops, out-and-backs, figure eights, or a combination of shapes.

Aerobic Difficulty On average, how out of breath you can expect to be; the scale ranges from 1 (super easy) to 5 (bring bottled oxygen).

Technical Difficulty On average, how tricky a particular ride is to negotiate due to terrain, traffic, and other variables; the scale ranges from 1 (look, no hands!) to 5 (bring the training wheels).

Scenery A short summary of what to expect in terms of plant life, wildlife, natural wonders, and historic features.

Exposure A quick check of how much sun you can expect on your shoulders during the ride. This book uses a "cooked meat" analogy for sun-exposure ratings: rare equals shady and cool; well-done equals plenty of sun; and so on.

Ride Traffic Indicates how busy the ride might be on an average day. Trail traffic, of course, varies from day to day and season to season. Weekends typically see more visitors.

Trail Surface Indicates whether the trail surface is paved, rocky, gravel, dirt, or a mixture of elements.

Riding Time The length of time it takes to complete the ride. My speed tends to be on the quick side, so I've used my numbers as the shorter time limit and allowed for a good amount of time for the upper time limit.

Access A notation of any fees or permits that may be needed to access the trail or park at the trailhead.

Maps The name(s) of relevant USGS topo maps and/or maps available at trailheads.

Facilities What to expect in terms of restrooms and water at the trailhead or nearby.

Directions

Used in conjunction with the overview map, the driving directions lead you to the trailhead. Once at the trailhead, park only in designated areas.

Weather

San Francisco is a very temperate city, if a little on the cold side. The temperature variances from day to night in the city are less severe than in the surrounding regions, which tend to get much warmer during the day in the summer and much colder at nights in the winter. The city is generally covered in fog but does not receive quite as much rain as do the regions beyond the bay. The wind tends to be much more severe in the city, though, and these winds can quickly turn a sunny day overcast and cold.

Average Temperature by Month (Fahrenheit)

	January	February	March	April	May	June
High	55	61	62	63	68	76
Low	45	47	50	51	53	68

	July	August	September	October	November	December
High	73	74	77	71	64	57
Low	56	55	56	56	50	45

Recreation happens year-round in the Bay Area, particularly in the areas close the city and coast, which rarely, if ever, see triple-digit temperatures. The East Bay often gets extremely warm in the summer, and that, combined with the severity of the terrain out that way, can make for a very sweaty ride. Even though temperatures allow for year-round riding, not all parks allow for wet-weather riding, and even if they do, different trail types have different resiliency. Following a rain, call ahead to find out if a park is open to riding, and even if the park is, make a judgment call as to whether or not you believe it is eco-sensible for you to be trekking through the mud.

Water

Always err on the side of excess when deciding how much water to pack: a rider working hard in a 90° heat needs about ten quarts of fluid per day. That's about 2.5 gallons. In other words, pack along one or two bottles even for short rides. For long rides, especially in hot weather, consider camelling water on your back in a hydration system.

Although the city of San Francisco gets its tap water from the Hetch Hetchy Reservoir, considered to be one of the cleanest (and tastiest) sources in the nation, most of the water you will come across on the rides in this book cannot be considered safe to drink. The threat of Giardia or poisoning from *E. coli* bacteria is just too great a risk in an area with this dense of a population, since the natural systems aren't capable of fully cleansing the amount of wastes that are effused.

Even where water is available, choosing to drink it comes with risks. Some riders are prepared to purify water found along the route. Purifiers with ceramic filters and charcoal pre-filters are the most efficient at weeding out bugs and chemicals. You can also pack along the slightly distasteful tetraglycine-hydroperiodide tablets to debug water (sold under names such as Potable Aqua and Coughlan's).

If you drink found water, the most common waterborne "bug" you'll face is Giardia, which may not hit until one to four weeks after ingestion. Giardia will have you living in the bathroom, passing noxious rotten-egg gas, vomiting, and shivering with chills. Other parasites to worry about include E. coli and cryptosporidium.

For most people, the pleasures of riding make carrying water a relatively minor price to pay to remain healthy. If you're tempted to drink found water, you should do so only if you understand the risks involved. Better yet, hydrate prior to your ride, carry (and drink) eight ounces of water for every mile you ride, and hydrate after the ride.

Clothing

Typical riding clothing is suitable for this area, although if you're riding near the coast or city center, you may wish to add an extra layer than what you would normally ride with. Always carry an additional layer with you because the temperature can drop rapidly in the region and being stuck on top of, say, Mount Diablo with a 25-minute cold descent ahead of you can get you very close to a case of hypothermia.

The Essentials

One of the first rules of riding is to be prepared for anything. The simplest way to be prepared is to carry the essentials. Always consider worst-case scenarios, such as getting lost, riding back in the dark, broken components, cranking a wrist, or a brutal thunderstorm. The items listed below don't cost a lot of money, don't take up much room in a pack, and don't weigh much—but they might just save your life.

- **Compass** (and GPS unit if you have one)
- **Extra clothes:** rain protection, warm layers, gloves, warm hat
- **Extra food:** you should always have some left when you've finished riding
- **Fire:** windproof matches or lighter and fire starter
- **First-aid kit:** a compact kit including first-aid instructions
- **Knife:** a bike multitool with a knife is best
- **Light:** flashlight or headlamp with extra bulbs and batteries
- **Map:** preferably a topo map and a copy of this book's trail map and ride description.
- **Mirror:** to attract attention from aircraft in emergencies
- **Sun protection:** sunglasses, lip balm, sunblock, sun hat (in case you have to walk)
- **Water:** durable bottles and water treatment such as iodine or a filter

Topo Maps

The maps in this book have been produced with great care and, used with the directions, will lead you to the trail and help you stay on course. However, you will find additional detail and valuable information in the United States Geological Survey's 7.5-minute series topographic maps. Topo maps are available online in many locations. The downside to USGS topos is that many of them are outdated, having been created 20 to 30 years ago.

Cultural features on outdated topo maps, such as roads, will probably be inaccurate, but the topographic features should be accurate.

Digital topographic map programs such as Delorme's TopoUSA enable you to review topo maps of the entire United States on your PC. Gathered while hiking with a GPS unit, GPS data can be downloaded onto the software and you can plot your own rides. Google Earth is a great free program that allows you to check aerial views of an area against a topo map.

If you're new to maps, you might be wondering what a topo map is. In short, a topo map indicates not only linear distance but elevation as well, using contour lines. Each brown squiggly line represents a particular elevation, and at the base of each topo a contour's interval designation is given. If the contour interval is 20 feet, then the distance between each contour line is 20 feet. Follow five contour lines up on the same map, and the elevation has increased by 100 feet. Every fifth contour line is labeled with an altitude. These lines are slightly heavier than the intervening contour lines and are called the index lines. An index line that reads "1,300" indicates a contour that is 1,300 feet above sea level.

In addition to the outdoor shops listed in the Appendix, you'll find topos at major universities and some public libraries, where you can photocopy the maps you need to avoid the cost of buying them. But if you want your own and can't find them locally, visit the United States Geological Survey Web site at **www.topomaps.usgs.gov.**

Also, don't overlook locally produced maps, which usually show superior detail for small areas. Examples include county road maps. Another reliable map source that contains updated road information on topo maps is DeLorme's *Gazetteer* series. There is a *Gazetteer* for each of the 50 U.S. states.

Bike Tools

Carrying these basics requires only a small seat bag or stem bag and is recommended even for short rides. In addition to carrying the items listed below, you need to know how to use them. The most common problem is probably the dreaded flat. If you opt for carrying only compressed air to reinflate tires, you run the risk of having more flats than you have air cylinders. A small collapsible pump solves that problem. Before you go, make sure your tire patch-kit's rubber cement hasn't dried out. If your chain snaps, you'll need a chain tool to piece it back together.

- Chain tool
- Duct tape
- Multitool
- Patch kit
- Spare tube
- Tire lever
- Tire pump and/or compressed air kit

The multitool should address the balance of repairs or adjustments (seat, brakes, derailleurs) you may need to make on a ride. If you snap your frame in half, just call it a day and don't bother with the tools.

First-aid Kit

A very basic first-aid kit may contain more items than you might think necessary. Prepackaged kits in waterproof bags are available (Atwater Carey and Adventure Medical make a variety of kits). Though quite a few items are listed here, they pack into a small space:

- Ace bandages for sprains or to make compression bandages
- Antibiotic ointment (Neosporin or the generic equivalent) for cuts
- Aspirin or acetaminophen for aches
- Band-Aids for cuts
- Benadryl or the generic equivalent diphenhydramine (in case of allergic reactions)
- Butterfly-closure bandages for deep cuts
- Epinephrine in a prefilled syringe (for people known to have severe allergic reactions to such things as bee stings)
- Gauze compress pads (a half dozen 4 x 4-inch pads) to clean and cover wounds
- Hydrogen peroxide or iodine for cuts and abrasions
- Insect repellent in case the bugs are on holiday
- Matches or pocket lighter to build fires for warmth, to heat water, or to cook food
- Roll of gauze to hold bandages on
- Sunscreen to prevent sunburn
- Whistle (it's more effective than your voice in signaling rescuers)

General Safety

Potentially dangerous situations can occur, but preparation and sound judgment result in safe forays into remote and wild areas. Here are a few tips to make your trip safer and easier.

- Make sure your car, truck, or SUV is in a good shape before you go to the park, and check road conditions before you set out. If your vehicle breaks down, stay with it—it's easier to find a vehicle than a person.
- Always carry food and water, whether you are planning an overnight trip or not. Food will give you energy, help keep you warm, and sustain you in an emergency situation until help arrives. Always bring water or boil/filter/treat found water before drinking it.
- Wear sturdy biking shoes
- Wear a professional-grade bike helmet (brain bucket)
- Never ride alone—take a buddy with you out on the trails
- Tell someone where you're going and when you'll be back (be as specific as possible), and ask him or her to get help if you don't return in a reasonable amount of time.

- Stay on the trails and routes described herein. Most riders get lost when they leave the path. Even on the most clearly marked trails, there is usually a point where you have to stop and consider which direction to head. If you become disoriented, don't panic. As soon as you think you may be off track, stop, assess your current direction, and then retrace your path back to the point where you went awry. Using a map, a compass, and this book, and keeping in mind what you have passed thus far, reorient yourself and trust your judgment on which way to continue. If you become absolutely unsure of how to proceed, return to your vehicle the way you came in. Should you become completely lost and have no idea of how to return to the trailhead, remaining in place along the trail and waiting for help is most often the best choice for adults and always the best option for kids. If you have prepared well, brought supplies, and taken that all-important step of telling someone where you'll be and for how long, staying in place shouldn't result in disaster.
- Take along your brain. A cool, calculating mind is the single most important piece of equipment you'll need on the trail. Think before you act. Watch your step. Plan ahead. Avoiding accidents before they happen is the best recipe for a rewarding and relaxing ride.
- Ask questions. It's a lot easier to get advice beforehand and avoid mishaps away from civilization, where finding help may be difficult. Use your head out there and treat the place as if it were your own backyard.

Animal and Plant Hazards

Ticks

Ticks are commonly found in brushy and woodsy areas. Ticks, which are arthropods and not insects, need a host to feast on in order to reproduce. The ticks that light onto you while riding will be very small, sometimes so tiny that you won't be able to spot them. Primarily of two varieties, deer ticks and dog ticks, they need a few hours of actual attachment before they can transmit any disease they may harbor. Ticks may settle in shoes, socks, or hats. The best strategy is to visually check every so often while riding; do a thorough check before you get in the car; and then, when you take a post-ride shower, do an even more thorough check of your entire body. Ticks that haven't attached are easily removed but not easily killed. If you pick off a tick while on the trail, just toss it aside. If you find one on your body at home, remove it and then send it down the toilet. For ticks that have embedded, removal with tweezers is best.

Snakes

In terms of venomous serpents, there are rattlesnakes and king snakes throughout the Bay Area. King snakes are rarely seen out in the open, but rattlesnakes can often be found sunning themselves on a trail or rock outcropping. The most prevalent large snake would have to be the gopher snake, which looks very similar to a rattlesnake and even mimics the rattling noise given off by a defensive rattlesnake. That said, I've never had an issue with snakes while on a mountain bike ride, only when hiking, which is one benefit of being elevated from the ground and moving quickly. The biggest danger comes when either you crash off the trail into the brush, or you stop to fix a flat. There's not much you can do to guard against snake bites in the event of a crash, but at least in the latter situation be cautious about where you set up to fix the flat. Snakes are more scared of us than we are of them—we just have to be careful not to get too close and elicit their defense responses.

Mountain Lions

Mountain lions can be found in many of the more remote parks and places in the Bay Area, and the explosion of development in the last couple of decades has forced the existing population into closer quarters with humans, which has led to a small number of sightings and an even smaller number of attacks. For the most part, this animal is as shy as any and doesn't want to have anything to do with an animal as weird and dangerous as the human. That said, any animal can be provoked, so follow good-sense guidelines for staying out of big cats' way.

Here are a few helpful guidelines for mountain-lion encounters:

- Keep kids close to you. Observed in captivity, mountain lions seem especially drawn to small children.
- Do not run from a mountain lion. Running may stimulate the animal's instinct to chase.
- Do not approach a mountain lion. Instead, give him room to get away.
- Try to make yourself look larger by raising your arms and/or opening your jacket if you're wearing one.
- Do not crouch or kneel down. These movements could make you look smaller and more like the lion's prey.
- Try to convince the lion you are dangerous—not its prey. Without crouching, gather nearby stones or branches and toss them at the animal. Slowly wave your arms above your head and speak in a firm voice.
- If all fails and you are attacked, fight back. People have successfully fought off an attacking lion with rocks and sticks. Try to remain facing the animal, and fend off its attempts to bite at your head or neck—a lion's typical aim.

Poison Oak

Poison oak is primarily recognized by its three-leaflet configuration—on either a vine or shrub. Usually within 12 to 14 hours of exposure (but sometimes much later), raised lines and/or blisters will appear, accompanied by a terrible itch. Urushiol, the oil in the sap of this plant, is responsible for the rash. Refrain from scratching, since bacteria under fingernails can cause infection; you can also spread the rash to other parts of your body by scratching. Wash and dry the rash thoroughly, applying a calamine lotion or other product to help dry the rash. If itching or blistering is severe, seek medical attention. Remember that oil-contaminated clothes, pets, or riding gear can easily cause an irritating rash on you or someone else, so be sure to wash exposed parts of your body, exposed clothes, gear, and pets.

Trail Etiquette

Whether you're on a city, county, state, or national park trail, always remember that great care and resources (from nature as well as from your tax dollars) have gone into creating these trails. Treat the trail, wildlife, and fellow riders with respect.

- Ride on open trails only. Respect trail and road closures (ask if not sure), avoid trespassing on private land, obtain permits and authorization as required, and leave gates as you found them or as marked.
- Leave only tire prints. Pack out what you pack in. No one likes to see the trash someone else has left behind.
- Never intentionally spook animals. An unannounced approach, a sudden movement, or a loud noise startles most animals. A surprised animal can be dangerous to you, to others, and to itself.
- Plan ahead. Know your bike, your ability, and the area in which you are riding—and prepare accordingly. Be self-sufficient at all times; carry necessary supplies for changes in weather or other conditions.
- Be courteous to other riders, riders, equestrians, and all others you encounter on the trails; maintaining a wide grin makes this task a lot easier.

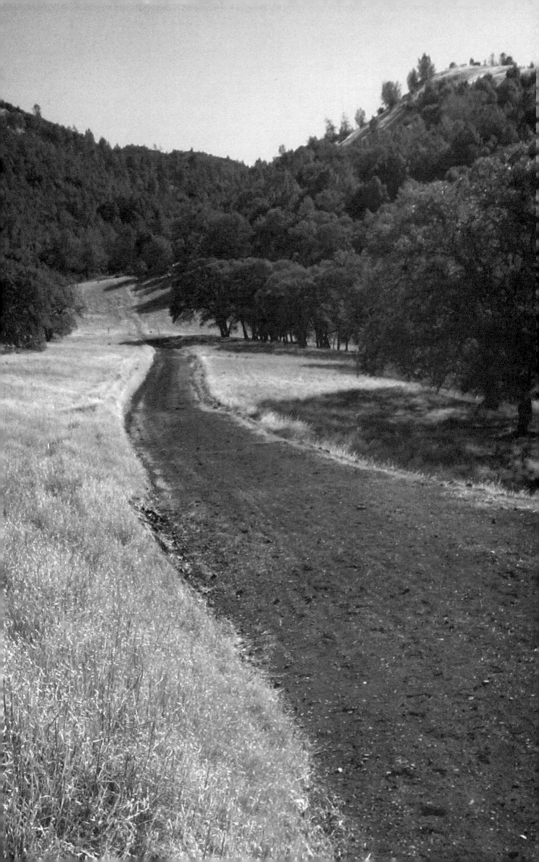

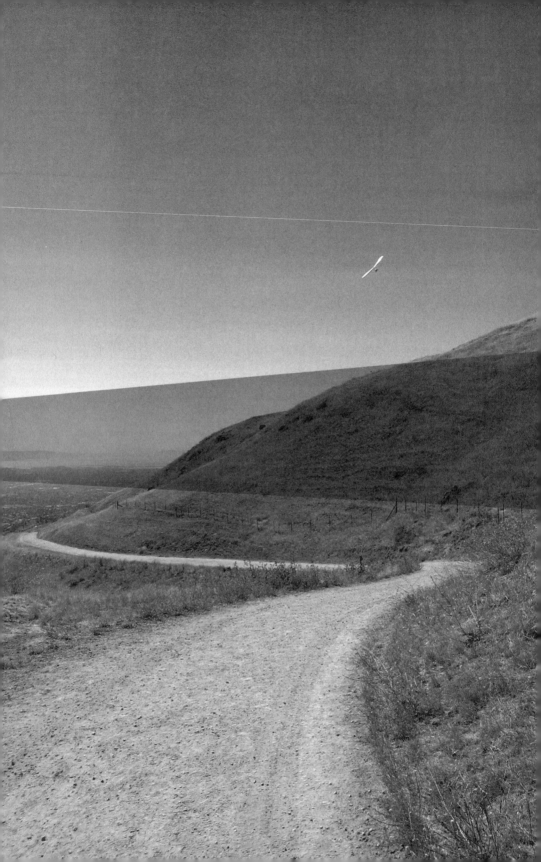

EAST BAY

WILDCAT CANYON REGIONAL PARK: HAVEY CANYON TO BELGUM TRAIL LOOP

KEY AT-A-GLANCE INFORMATION

Length: 11.28 miles

Configuration: Loop with 2.6-mile out-and-back

Difficulty: 5/10; a perfect blend

Scenery: Commanding views of San Francisco Bay

Exposure: Well-done

Ride traffic: High, because this park's in the middle of everything

Riding time: 1.75–2.5 hours

Access: Free parking

Facilities: Water fountains and restrooms in parking lot

In Brief

It's hard to believe that a park as big as Wildcat Canyon can exist right smack in the middle of such a heavily developed region as the Bay Area. This ride takes you up Havey Canyon singletrack (so good you'll want to descend and climb it again), out along the San Pablo Ridge, and down the Belgum Wall, for just over 11 miles of moderately challenging riding. This park is such a great asset to Bay Area mountain bikers—now if we can just get a continuous bike lane across the Bay Bridge, we'll be set.

Contact

Wildcat Canyon Regional Park
5755 McBryde Avenue
Richmond, CA 94506
(510) 236-1262; www.ebparks.org/parks/wildcat

DIRECTIONS

By bike: From San Francisco, take the Richmond train and get off at the North Berkeley stop. Head north out of the station and make your first right onto Virginia Street. Ride through six four-way intersections east on Virginia Street until you come to Shattuck Avenue, where you make a left. Ride four blocks north on Shattuck Avenue and make a right onto Rose Street. Ride three blocks and make a left onto Spruce Street, which is a strenuous climb up onto the hill. At the top of the hill, find Canon Drive at the far end of a complicated intersection, descend into the park, and follow the signs that say "Bike Access to Wildcat."

By car: From San Francisco, drive east across the Bay Bridge and follow Interstate 80 East toward Sacramento. Exit I-80 at Buchanan Street toward Albany; this street will change into Marin Avenue, which you'll take for 1.9 miles and then turn left onto Spruce Street, which will take you to the top of the hill. Find Canon Drive at the far end of a complicated intersection and descend down into the park. At the bottom of the hill, make a right and then take the first left onto Lone Oak Road.

GPS TRAILHEAD COORDINATES (WGS 84)

UTM Zone 10S
Easting 0564950
Northing 4195640
Latitude N 37° 54' 28.1"
Longitude W 122° 15' 40.1"

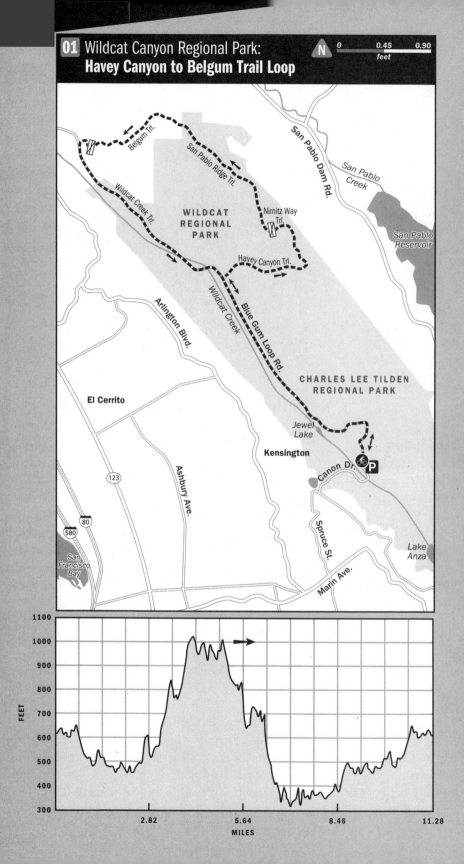

N

0   0.45   0.90
feet

WILDCAT
REGIONAL
PARK

Belgum Trl.

San Pablo Ridge Trl.

San Pablo Dam Rd.

San Pablo Creek

San Pablo Reservoir

Nimitz Way Trl.

Wildcat Creek Trl.

Havey Canyon Trl.

Arlington Blvd.

Wildcat Creek

Blue Gum Loop Rd.

CHARLES LEE TILDEN
REGIONAL PARK

El Cerrito

Jewel Lake

Kensington

Ashbury Ave.

Canon Dr.

P

123

80

580

San Francisco Bay

Spruce St.

Marin Ave.

Lake Anza

FEET

1100
1000
900
800
700
600
500
400
300

2.82   5.64   8.46   11.28
MILES

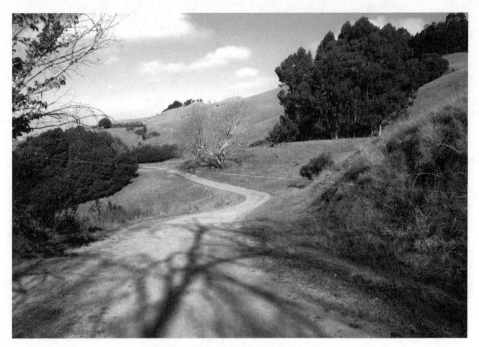

View at the bottom of Belgum Trail

Description

The ride actually begins at the Lone Oak picnic area off Lone Oak Road in Tilden Regional Park, which borders Wildcat Canyon Regional Park to the south. Should you ever want to explore Tilden Park, there are two additional trailheads located here that lead into Tilden Park: Wildcat Gorge Trail and Meadows Canyon Trail, both of which are mountain bike legal. Today's trail, Blue Gum Loop Road, continues where Lone Oak Road leaves off at the Blue Gum campground; pass through the gate, where the pavement ends and the dirt begins.

Blue Gum Loop Road is a fire road that climbs slightly for the first quarter mile, riding through a forest of eucalyptus trees past various campgrounds and no-bikes singletracks, and then turns into a mellow descent down to Jewel Lake. This lake is incredibly scenic, and you'll regularly see ducks and turtles on the rocks basking in the sun, so you may want to plan for a stop off here, either on the way out or on the way back, since you will pass back by this way. There are restrooms and water fountains here as well.

Beyond the lake, Blue Gum Loop Road changes names to Wildcat Creek Trail, which you'll often find roughed up by the tire tracks of park vehicles that have driven through the mud. Three-quarters of a mile past the lake you'll see a sign declaring your entrance into Wildcat Canyon. The trees recede, opening up views to the ridges on either side of you; on the left ridge you can spot a few of the large homes perched above the hillside covered in oaks. The right hillside is more grassland, with a few clusters of oaks, primarily gathered in the water-rich crevices. Tunnels are occasionally formed where the dense, shrubby vegetation that runs alongside much of the trail actually begins to overwhelm it.

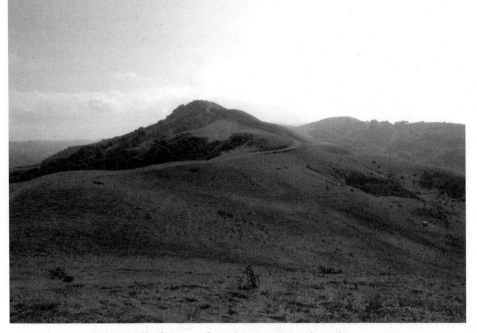

You'll often see fog whipping over the ridge.

At the next major intersection of fire roads, 2.6 miles into the ride, make a right onto Havey Canyon Trail/Conlon Trail and immediately make a left to stay on Havey Canyon Trail, which shortly turns into singletrack. This is a special trail because it is one of the few multiuse singletracks in all of the East Bay parks system that is open to mountain bikes, with the only restriction being that mountain bikes cannot be on the trail in wet conditions.

Trail-use politics aside, Havey Canyon is just a fantastic trail—a tree-shrouded, twisty singletrack that follows the small valley up the hillside. Belgum Trail, which comes later in the ride, is the real reason that this ride is done in a counterclockwise fashion, but Havey Canyon Trail is a lot of fun in both directions, and, as was mentioned above, you'll probably want to turn right around at the top and descend down, just to climb it again. About midway up this 1.3-mile climb, the trail crosses a creek, and it's a crossing that cannot be ridden due to the depth and angle of this bedrock waterway. Even if you've got serious trials skills, the slickness of the rocks will lead to your undoing, so just portage it. The positive aspect of this short section is that horses would be completely unable to make it across, and it keeps equestrians off this gem until they fix it. Let's just hope they don't ever fix it.

Toward the top, Havey Canyon Trail exits the trees and the trail gets uncharacteristically rough, with a slathering of small potholes. You'll pass through a self-closing gate and ride about 130 yards up to where the trail Ts into paved Nimitz Way; make a left here. Nimitz Way climbs the last little bit up onto the ridge, and the pavement only lasts for about half a mile before veering left and turning into to dirt and then shortly changing into Mezue Trail.

You're gonna want to follow San Pablo Ridge Trail along the ridge, so avoid Old Nimitz Way, which peels off to the right, and Mezue Trail, which peels off to the left. Fortunately, if the geographic nature of this trail eludes you, the signage here is good and will provide you with direction. The top of the mountain is bare of trees, and on a clear day you'll get views all around, from San Pablo Reservoir to the east, to San Francisco to the west. There are a few benches placed along the ridge should you care to stop and take it all in.

You'll pass a stable actively used for the cattle that graze this park and will climb steeply up to the 1,057-foot peak. Descend down the other side of the peak, taking care not to run into bovine obstacles of any sort, ride out to the far end of the ridge, and make a left onto Belgum Trail. As you spin along this fire road you'll often scare up a number of birds that nest in the grass.

Belgum Trail is steep, with one section in particular that hits 18 percent, and for this reason it's preferable to descend rather than climb this trail. The steepest bit is really the only problem on this fun descent—it tends to be chewed up and rough, but the visibility is good, so you'll be able to see other users ahead of time and moderate your approach accordingly. The lower portion of the trail winds through a series of oak, eucalyptus, and palm trees before hitting a gate at the very bottom. At this point the trail is comprised of some neglected, old pavement. Make a left onto Wildcat Creek Trail, which is also cracked pavement, and ride south. The pavement only lasts three-fourths of a mile before turning back into dirt, and then it's one relatively flat mile to the intersection with Havey Canyon Trail, at which point you'll just backtrack past Jewel Lake back to the car.

After the Ride

When you make your way back into town, you have a number of great eating options, from taco trucks to Gordo's burritos (a great Bay Area chain) to fine dining to college-student favorites such as Raleigh's. For a sit-down meal in a casual atmosphere, check out El Sombero Taqueria on the corner of University Avenue and Shattuck, just a few blocks from the Downtown Berkeley BART stop. The burritos are gigantic, so if you did opt to ride Havey Canyon Trail a few extra times, you'll be able to get the needed caloric replacement here. Call (510) 843-1311 for more information.

02

REDWOOD REGIONAL PARK: BIG LOOP PLUS GRAHAM AND DUNN

KEY AT-A-GLANCE INFORMATION

Length: 9.94 miles

Configuration: Counterclockwise loop

Difficulty: 8/10; more than 2,500 feet of climbing!

Scenery: Two sides of the same canyon, and the Chabot Space and Science Center

Exposure: Medium-well

Ride traffic: High. Due to the ease of access from the surrounding townships, you'll generally find a large number of people enjoying this park.

Riding time: 2–3 hours

Access: $5 parking fee

Facilities: Restrooms and water fountains at the start and middle-point of the ride

In Brief

A slight deviation from the recommended Redwood Bike Loop indicated in the park brochure, this loop adds the Graham-and-Dunn-trails combination on the west ridge and is the largest contiguous bike-accessible loop on offer in Redwood Park.

Contact

Redwood Regional Park
7867 Redwood Road
Oakland, CA 94619
(510) 562-7275
www.ebparks.org/parks/redwood

Description

Locate Canyon Trail to the right of the parking lot entrance. Slip your tires onto the dirt and ride up past the picnic benches and into the woods. Once the trail turns right into the woods, it pitches up sharply. The climb follows a small streambed on the left shaded primarily by bay trees, which abandon you after the first 280 yards, leaving the last 280 yards of the climb up onto the ridge exposed, surrounded by chaparral.

Once on top of the ridge, Canyon Trail Ts into East Ridge Trail. Make a left to head northwest on East Ridge Trail. You gain 300 feet in elevation very quickly to bring

GPS TRAILHEAD COORDINATES (WGS 84)

UTM Zone 10S
Easting 0575060
Northing 4184520
Latitude N 37° 48' 24.4"
Longitude W 122° 8' 49.6"

DIRECTIONS

Take Interstate 80 East out of the city, across the Bay Bridge toward Oakland. Merge onto Interstate 580 toward Oakland/Stockton. Drive 6.3 mile on I-580 and take the 35th Avenue exit. Turn left onto 35th Avenue and follow that to where it turns into Redwood Road. Take Redwood Road 3.9 miles to Redwood Gate, make a left, and enter the park.

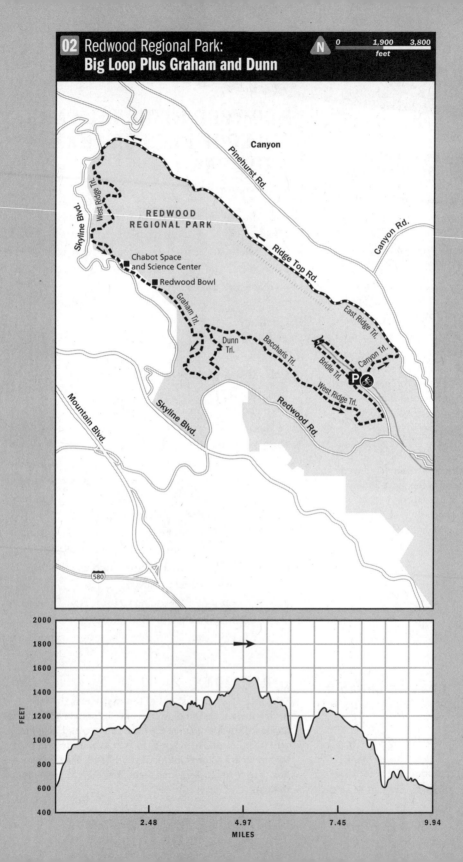

N   0   1,900   3,800
                 feet

Canyon

Pinehurst Rd.

Canyon Rd.

Skyline Blvd.

West Ridge Trl.

REDWOOD
REGIONAL PARK

Chabot Space
and Science Center

Redwood Bowl

Graham Trl.

Dunn
Trl.

Bacharis Trl.

East Ridge Trl.

Canyon Trl.

Bridle Trl.

P

West Ridge Trl.

Mountain Blvd.

Skyline Blvd.

Redwood Rd.

580

2000
1800
1600
1400
1200
1000
800
600
400

FEET

2.48   4.97   7.45   9.94
MILES

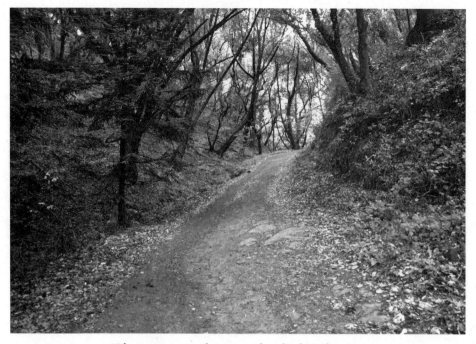

When you enter the trees, the climbing begins.

you up onto the ridge, but once up there, the climbing evens out, and you roll along the top of the ridge on a broad fire road surrounded mostly by coyote brush. The trail surface is mostly smooth but can be rough following storms when horse hooves have pitted the trail surface.

Gradually the chaparral gives way to pine trees, affording some shade on hot days. There aren't any intersecting trails until mile 2.1, when Prince Road shoots off to the left, but this is a no-bikes trail and well marked as such. In fact, all of the trails in the valley are off-limits to bikes, so ignore all such trails and keep your focus on East Ridge Trail, which will terminate at the Skyline Gate parking lot.

Skyline Gate parking lot is probably the most popular access point to the park, and it is a good option for starting this ride. There are portable toilets and water fountains here.

Skirt the parking lot and find West Ridge Trail where it begins at the west side of the lot. As soon as you lay tire on this trail, you realize that west is better than east when it comes to Redwood Regional Park. West Ridge Trail is a mildly rocky doubletrack that winds through eucalyptus, bay, pine, and madrona trees, through which you get incredibly reward-ing glimpses to the other side of the canyon.

The trail begins climbing again, but not drastically, averaging just a 5 percent gradient. Just as with the other side of the park, most of the little splinter trails are closed to bikes, indicated with the typical signs featuring a poorly rendered bicycle behind a red circle-slash.

The park's name contains the word *redwood*, but it isn't until mile 3.8 of this ride that you actually see any up close, as they're all tucked away in the northwest corner of the park.

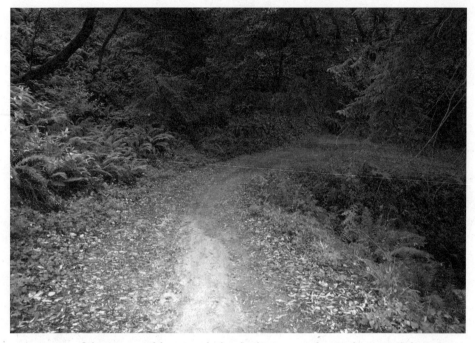

Just one of the impeccably smooth, banked turns on the Graham Trail descent

The trail continues as doubletrack, winding along over the occasional section of bedrock peaking through the dirt and roughing things up a tad.

A brief descent brings you to Moon Gate on the right, which is another access point to the park, leading out to Skyline Boulevard. The trail then climbs for another 45 yards before coming to a gate and a paved road. Up this road you find the Chabot Space and Science Center, which is only partially visible from the trail. Cross the road to where the trail resumes on the other side and watch to your left as some large gray and silver buildings loom large on the hill above you, nestled in with the trees. The buildings are constructed of cement, polished aluminum, and glass and make use of spherical and angular shapes to fantastic effect; it's really an otherworldly sight.

The space center also marks the peak elevation on this ride at 1,530 feet, 4.8 miles into the ride. From here the trail descends slightly for a third of a mile, picking its way through redwood trees, and then comes to a four-way intersection. Left takes you to the archery range, while right takes you down the Redwood Bowl Staging Area. Head straight, continuing on West Ridge Trail toward Redwood Bowl, which you reach in another 110 yards.

Redwood Bowl is aptly named, being about the size of a football field, slightly concave, and surrounded by tall redwoods. This is a great place to stop for a snack, and you often see picnickers here enjoying the provided picnic facilities (tables, BBQ pits, and water fountains).

About 18 yards beyond the bowl, West Ridge Trail intersects with Graham Trail. Turn right onto Graham Trail and get ready to descend. This doubletrack plummets through the trees, alternating between shaded and exposed sections, and passes over a number of rocky and/or washboard-laden sections, all of which combine to make this an Anne-Caroline Chausson–worthy descent. Along this descent, Roberts Park Trail intersects from the right on two occasions, but other than that there are no forks, so just keep it in your mind to stay left, and you'll stay on Graham Trail.

After descending for nearly a mile, Graham Trail terminates into Dunn Trail. Going right on Dunn Trail would take you down to Redwood Road in just over a mile, and that could be another option for a starting point for this loop. However, take the left at this junction and follow Dunn Trail back into the park.

Dunn Trail ceases the descending for the moment, offering a rolling 1.1-mile climb up to the next major junction with Baccharis Trail. The unmarked trail that appears on the right 0.8 miles up this climb is Monteiro Trail, a fun descent that terminates at Redwood Road; ignore this and proceed to the left on Dunn Trail.

The merger with Baccharis Trail, a doubletrack that approaches from behind and to the left, is marked by the sandy trail conditions. The trail passes through a meadow, and the sand does its best to slow you down, but you're aided by the fact that the remainder of the ride is descent. At mile 7.5 West Ridge Trail reemerges on the left, and Baccharis Trail smoothly integrates into its southeastern direction.

The descent continues mildly for the next 0.75 miles, cutting along the ridge with great views on both sides, but you're still up above 1,000 feet—remember that the parking lot is down at 600 feet. When you see the sign stating DOWN GRADE; REDUCE SPEED, you know where that last 400 feet is going to come from.

This is a great descent, very much in the vein of the Graham Trail descent, but even steeper, and thus faster. There are some rough spots and a few good switchbacks, one of which features a wall ride with a three-foot-high apex.

At the bottom, make a left onto Bridle Trail, a smooth, flat promenade lined with an old wooden fence that cuts along the creek at the base of the canyon. Make a right where the trail hits the pavement and follow the signs back to the Canyon Bike Loop—this will lead you back to the parking lot.

After the Ride

Get back on Redwood Road/35th Avenue, heading west back toward town. Pass under I-580, drive 1.75 miles to International Boulevard, and make a left. Drive one and half blocks south on International Boulevard to find Taqueria El Farolito at 3646 International Boulevard. This place has excellent and inexpensive super burritos, and a menu full of other delicious authentic Mexican food, as well as *agua fresca*. Call (510) 533-9194 for more information.

LAKE CHABOT REGIONAL PARK: LAKE CHABOT BICYCLE LOOP

KEY AT-A-GLANCE INFORMATION

Length: 10.7 miles

Configuration: Counterclockwise loop

Difficulty: 7/10; steep climb up from the lake; long loop

Scenery: Eucalyptus and redwood forests, beautiful small lake

Exposure: Medium

Ride traffic: Marina is crowded, but only mild traffic in back two-thirds of the park

Riding time: 1.75–2.5 hours

Access: $5 parking fee in Lake Chabot parking lot but lots of free parking along Lake Chabot Avenue

Facilities: Restrooms, water fountains, and barbecues

In Brief

An enjoyable East Bay fire-road loop starting and ending at the Lake Chabot Marina. The marina is a lively place on nice days and a great place for a picnic. Those of your party not inclined to undertake the moderately arduous Lake Chabot Bicycle Loop (such as your kids or not-into-mountain-biking friends, etc.) can find plenty to do around the marina while you head up into the hills in search of this park's mythical eucalyptus forest.

Contact

Lake Chabot Regional Park
17600 Lake Chabot Road
Castro Valley, CA 94546
(888) 327-2757
www.ebparks.org/parks/lake_chabot

Description

The 315-acre Lake Chabot was created by Anthony Chabot in 1879, and gradually, throughout the next 80 years,

GPS TRAILHEAD COORDINATES (WGS 84)

UTM Zone 10S
Easting 0579200
Northing 4174500
Latitude N 37° 42' 57.3"
Longitude W 122° 6' 4.4"

DIRECTIONS

By car: From San Francisco, take the Bay Bridge east over the bay and merge onto Interstate 580 East toward Hayward/Stockton. Drive approximately 14 miles to exit 32, which you will take toward Fairmont Drive. Merge onto Freedom Avenue and turn left onto Fairmont Drive. In 2 miles make a right onto Lake Chabot Road. Proceed for 0.3 miles past the park, which is on your left beyond a center divide. Make a U-turn and return to the park.

By public transportation/bike: Take the Dublin/Pleasanton BART train to the Castro Valley stop. Exit the station and get on Redwood Road, which is a large road running perpendicular to the train. Ride north on Redwood Road a half mile to Somerset Avenue and make a left. Take Somerset Avenue to Lake Chabot Road and make a right. Ride 1.5 miles to the park entrance.

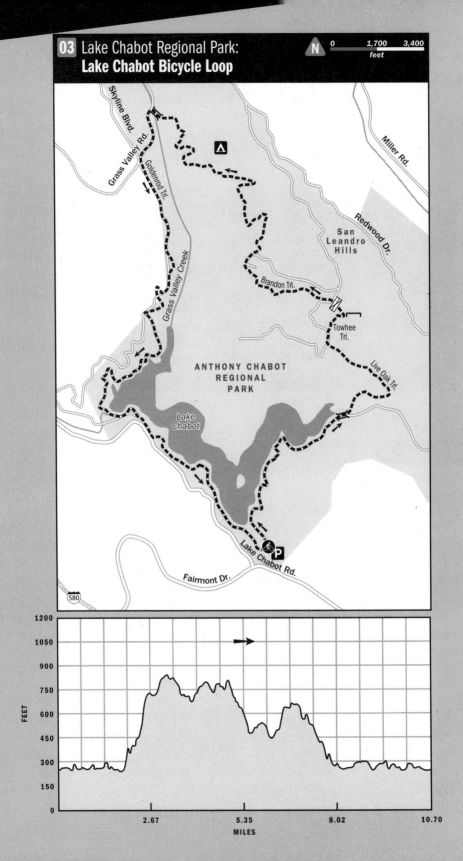

N

0   1,700   3,400
feet

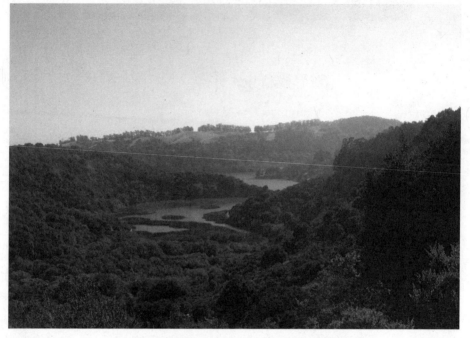

A view of Lake Chabot from Live Oak Trail

a total of 1,178 surrounding acres were leased by the park district to create the park as we know it today. Geographically this park runs northwest and connects successively with Anthony Chabot Regional Park and Redwood Regional Park, addressed elsewhere in this book.

Starting at the main park information sign at the base of the marina parking lot, head past the sign on the paved trail. On a sunny day, this park can be bustling with barbecuers, birthday party–goers, anglers, walkers, and joggers. It's far enough from the highfalutin hustle of the central Bay Area, though, and most people at Lake Chabot seem a little bit nicer and more inclined to say hi. From the sign it's just a 100 feet to the lake, and when you come to it, make a right so that the lake will be on your left.

To get to the actual trail, you've got to ride 1.8 miles along the paved path running along the lake. It's a crowded path, but a great way to get your legs warmed up. You'll come to an open gate and a sign announcing the Lake Chabot Bicycle Loop (LCBL), both of which signal the start of the dirt. The *start of the dirt* also signals the start of the dirt, but it's good to talk about landmarks. Ahem.

Head just 0.1 mile down the fire road and look for another of the LCBL signs on your left. Below this sign is a really cool 33-yard-long, 1-yard-wide footbridge that you must cross to get into the backwoods proper. The rules indicate that you have to walk your bike across the bridge; there are steps down to the bridge, and it's so narrow that it would be prohibitive to even try riding across. It really is a cool, bouncy little bridge over a lush, marshy terrain, but it's a wonder they didn't make it just a tad wider as it's difficult to pass people with bike in hand. The bridge landing on the other side is a particularly scenic spot, so be sure to turn around and have a look.

As you come to a four-way intersection, head straight onto Live Oak Trail. There is another large sign here describing the LCBL. It says it's a 12.42-mile loop, but somehow in the times that I've ridden it, I've never managed to find the extra 1.7 miles that I seem to be missing. It's a mystery to me.

Hopefully your legs are warm because you're about to climb almost straight up the hillside for the next 1.25 miles. It seems that the Switchback Construction Crew was on strike the day they made this section of trail, because there is nothing easy about this climb up the rutted, dusty fire road. Don't worry; the rest of the ride certainly isn't like this. Despite the huffing and puffing, try, if you can, to enjoy the pretty live oaks and chaparral that surround you.

As you come up onto the ridge, you get great views down to the lake on your left, and just a bit higher you can see across the rolling green hills to Castro Valley. At the next fork, make a right onto Towhee Trail, which follows a paved road for a few yards before veering away to the right. There are a few clusters of pretty wildflowers growing in this section all through spring and into early summer.

Go left at the next fork, but not onto the no-bikes singletrack. Or you can stop and take a break at the bench here and take in some food and views.

At mile 3.25 you'll come to a gate. Pass through the gate and cross the paved road. Following the crosswalk across the road takes you directly to another LCBL sign and Brandon Trail.

Brandon Trail starts out on a slight downhill and offers up more narrow fire road, but this time with the added twist of washboard. You chatter down through a grassy meadow before entering a small, enchanting stand of eucalyptus. It's very pretty in this section, especially late in the day when the light comes through the trees in diagonal shafts. When the poison oak in this area starts changing colors, it adds a whole new dimension.

The trail flattens out and then comes to a fork. This fork is Logger's Loop, and it connects with the trail here and in another 0.6 miles. Make a right at both occasions, staying on Brandon Trail, unless you care to make a walking detour down Logger's Loop.

Brandon Trail starts to pitch up and enters another, larger eucalyptus forest. This particular eucalyptus forest has an eerie feel to it: as you are cranking silently (well, maybe silently) up the hill, you can here the eucalyptus branches rubbing against each other as the trees are swayed by the wind. They do a good enough job of blocking the wind that it is virtually silent except for the high-pitched creaking noise the branches make. The leaves and bark shed by these trees cover the ground, and their smell infuses the air, all of which contribute to earning this trail an "awesome" rating.

Make a right and a straight at the next two forks, respectively, continuing on Brandon Trail. After the second fork, the trail makes a fun rocky descent down through the eucalyptus before it kicks back up again and passes between two small electrical towers.

Turn left at the next fork, staying on Brandon Trail, which is well marked as LCBL. There is ample signage throughout the park, indicating everything from trail name to trail etiquette, such as the sign at the top of the next extended downhill, which reads: BEGIN DOWNGRADE, REDUCE SPEED, CALL OUT. Always good advice when descending in a popular park. On this downhill you'll find that some pine and bay trees have joined in the eucalyptus party, and the resulting visual of wildly intersecting branches and differing green hues is nice.

At the bottom of the descent, at mile 6, make a left at the fork and cross the rock bridge (this one you can ride across). Across the bridge is another LCBL sign, directing you to go left onto Goldenrod Trail, where you'll climb up through a small grove of young redwood trees.

A trail splits right and behind at the next fork, but ignore it because you just want to stay on Goldenrod Trail. There is a paved road to your right, and the intersection of Skyline and Grass Valley roads is visible. Riding along this ridge, you can see left across the small valley to the trail you were just on. Ride through an open grassland with a lot of pretty thistles blooming purple in the summer.

Continue on Goldenrod Trail through the next fork. Columbine Trail runs left, but it is hiking only. Riding along, suddenly the trail makes a sharp downhill right turn, and the lake dramatically comes back into view after hiding from you in the hills for the last 6 miles. It's a pretty view, albeit somewhat obscured by the power lines running right through here. The trail then dips back into the trees for a fast washboard descent.

Strike pavement, go back 20 spaces. Just kidding. Go left and ride the pavement for about 55 yards (it's just a golf cart path that joins Goldenrod Trail for a short stretch). Make a left off the pavement at the weirdest yellow diamond sign I've ever seen on a trail: there's a squiggly arrow at the top—OK, meandering trail; that's obvious enough. But below that there are a lone stick-figure hiker on the left, a stick-figure hiking duo on the right, and a stick figure cyclist, all heading toward the left corner of the sign without any sort of symbolism relating them to each other. I've puzzled over this thing for awhile and still can't understand its meaning. Ride 100 feet to the next fork and make a left (yet another sign indicates that right is a restricted area).

The next sign points left to Bass Cove and right to the marina, 2.8 miles. Turning right brings you right down onto the water's edge, and it's an idyllic spot set in the trees. Make a right and a left through the next two forks, ride 30 feet and cross a paved path, and then make a left onto the next paved path you come to. Sorry, but that's the end of the dirt. First thing you come to is the dam. Apparently, Anthony Chabot created the dam by having workers dump bucketfuls of dirt and then herding wild stallions back and forth across the dam to pack it down. That sounds both grueling and interesting. Well, it's not nearly as interesting today. In fact it's quite boring and uninviting due to the tall chain-link fences running high along either side. Ride a little more than a mile back to the marina and unpack the picnic.

After the Ride

Try Genghis Khan Kitchen at 20855 Redwood Road, just a block and a half from the BART station. This place has a great Chinese food buffet and even some sushi options, which should fill you up after a long ride around the Lake Chabot Bicycle Loop. Call (510) 537-3862 for more information.

BRIONES REGIONAL PARK: MOTT PEAK LOOP

Length: 6.23 miles

Configuration: Clockwise loop

Difficulty: 3/10; short, with only 1,400 feet of climbing

Scenery: The intersection of Abrigo and Briones Crest trails is visually exquisite.

Exposure: Medium

Ride traffic: High on weekday afternoon/evenings and weekends

Riding time: 1–1.75 hours

Access: $5 parking fee at Bear Creek Staging Area

Facilities: Restrooms and water

In Brief

Framed by four of the major freeways that define the East Bay, near the ever-expanding bedroom communities of Orinda, Lafayette, and Walnut Creek, the bounding green hills of Briones Regional Park are your place to escape after trudging home through that five o' clock sea of red brake lights. Beginning at the Bear Creek Staging Area, this loop makes a circuit around Mott Peak, the tallest hill in the park, and is a great introduction to what is on offer here. As you become more familiar with the park, you can create many varying loops and also find some of the other access points that are hidden in the back of the surrounding neighborhoods.

Contact

Briones Regional Park
2537 Reliez Valley Road
Martinez, CA 94553
(925) 370-3020; www.ebparks.org/parks/briones

DIRECTIONS

By car: From San Francisco, head east across the Bay Bridge on Interstate 80. Once across the bridge, take the Interstate 580 East exit toward downtown Oakland/Hayward-Stockton/CA 24 and immediately take the CA 24/Grover Shafter Freeway East exit toward Walnut Creek. Drive almost 9 miles and exit on Acalanes Road/Mount Diablo Boulevard. Drive under the freeway, make a right onto El Nido Ranch Road, and then take a quick left onto Upper Happy Valley Road. Take this to where it intersects Happy Valley Road and make a left. Take Happy Valley Road up and over the ridge to where it Ts into Bear Creek Road and make a right. Drive half a mile up Bear Creek Road and find the entrance to Briones Regional Park on your right.

By public transportation: From San Francisco, take the Pittsburg/Bay Point BART train to the Lafayette stop. Ride through the parking lot to Deer Hill Road and make a left. Ride 0.25 miles down Deer Hill Road and make a right onto Happy Valley Road, then follow the directions above.

GPS TRAILHEAD COORDINATES (WGS 84)

UTM Zone 10S
Easting 0574080
Northing 4197880
Latitude N 37° 55' 38.8"
Longitude W 122° 9' 25.3"

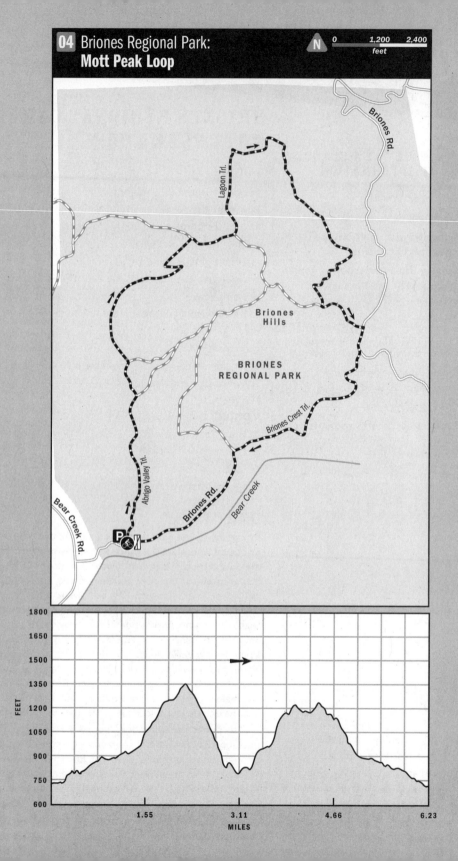

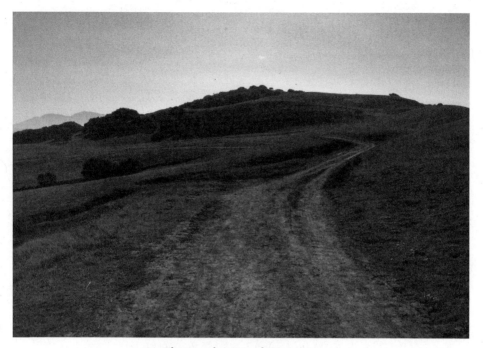

The run down to the Lagoon

Description

If you live anywhere in the vicinity of this park, chances are it has already infused itself into your life and you are probably aware of the many semihidden access points along the southern and eastern sides of the park (that is, close to CA 4 and Interstate 680). One of the joys of learning this park is discovering these hidden entrances from the inside out by exploring every trail to its genesis. If you're traveling to the park from a distance, though, it's much easier to park at one of the staging areas, such as Bear Creek. This straightforward loop starts from Bear Creek Staging Area on the western edge of the park, farthest from the freeways and suburbs. It's a great introduction to the park and offers many opportunities to add flower petals and extend the mileage by a little or a lot.

From Bear Creek Road, take the right onto Briones Road, well marked with a Briones Regional Park sign, and after paying at the parking kiosk, park in the first parking lot on the left. The Abrigo Valley Trailhead is located at the mouth of the parking lot on your right as you drive/ride in. It begins as a gravel road running through a broad meadow known as the Oak Grove picnic area, at the far end of which you'll find a self-closing cattle gate nestled in the trees. Pass through the gate and enter the park proper.

Abrigo Valley Trail, like all but a couple of the bike-legal trails in the park, is a fire road, and it climbs gradually up through the shallow, oak tree–filled valley. Just under a mile in, you come to the first intersection with Mott Peak Trail; make a left. Mott Peak Trail is a popular trail to descend in the other direction. Continue up Abrigo Valley Trail, passing by

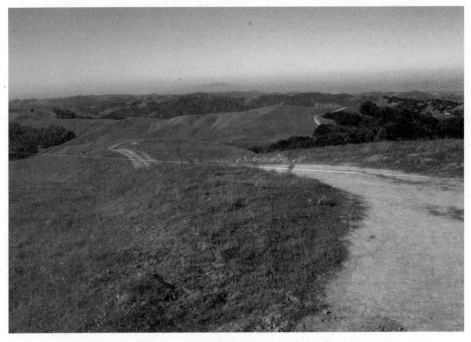

**Fire Road snaking along the hilltops away from the intersection
of Abrigo Valley and Briones Crest trails**

the Maud Whalen campground. The trail wraps to the right around the base of Mott Peak, passing by Santos Trail on the left, to where the valley terminates in the crux of the hills. Here is the first of two leg-breaking climbs on this loop.

This climb goes up a couple of switchbacks and up the spine of the hill, gaining 350 feet in elevation in a third of a mile, and plops you on the top of the ridge where Abrigo Valley Trail Ts into Briones Crest Trail. Traction is generally very good, as the trail is compacted, but it can be rough as the combination of cows' and horses' hooves, as well as ranger vehicles, chew up the trail surface when muddy and leave behind a jarring texture when it dries.

On the treeless ridge, the intersection of Abrigo Valley and Briones Crest trails features incredible panoramic views. Here you can see all of the surrounding hills and trace the various trails of the park as they splinter off in all directions, light brown lines slicing through green hills. On a clear day you can see Briones Reservoir to the west.

Make a right onto Briones Crest Trail and ride 0.25 miles along the ridge to Lagoon Trail, where you make a left. Lagoon Trail is a fun descent down the backside of Briones Crest on one of the finger ridges. It's a treeless descent with good visibility. Of course, due to the cattle grazing in the park, and the extra bovine trail traffic this creates, you need to be extra careful on descents.

Where the trail dives right off the small finger ridge, ignore the unmarked trail that splits off to the left—it just leads to the park boundary. The trail bottoms out after a broad zigzag and then enters the trees, rolling along for half a mile, passing by Toyon

Canyon Trail. If you want to drastically expand the loop, you can take the left on Toyon Canyon Trail and piece together a number of the trails in the eastern side of the park—but for now continue on Lagoon Trail.

Just 220 yards past the junction with Toyon Canyon Trail, Lagoon Trail makes an ominous right turn and points you up the hillside for a grueling 14 percent climb back up onto the ridge. Traction is similar to the earlier climb up to Briones Crest Trail, if not even a little more rough due to the higher cattle traffic in this area. At the top of the climb, the trail passes by the bigger of the two Sindicich Lagoons just before meeting back up with Briones Crest Trail, the other side of which is the smaller Sindicich Lagoon. The lagoons are fenced-off wildlife habitats, surrounded by reeds and partially covered in floating algae, but aside from the occasional dragonflies and birds, they aren't all that much to look at.

Make the sharp left at the little lagoon onto Briones Crest Trail and ride past a well-used water trough, 0.25 miles to Old Briones Road. Turn right onto Old Briones Road, which doubles up with Briones Crest Trail for a stone's throw to where the trails diverge; Briones Crest Trail continues up the hill and Old Briones Road passes through a gate and heads down the hill. Take the latter option, and as you pass through the gate, the valley is spread before you, with Mott Peak on your right and Old Briones Road cutting along the opposite hillside.

The top of the descent is steep and curvy, and a little on the rough side. The trail flattens out considerably where two valleys converge at the intersection of Old Briones and Valley trails; turn right to keep on Old Briones Road. At the end of a large plain, 5.3 miles into the ride, you come to the junction with Black Oak Trail. Continuing down Old Briones Road would bring you back to the parking lot in just under a mile; just head straight until you get to the pavement. However, a popular addition to this loop is to make the right onto Black Oak Trail, which is a fairly steep but technically entertaining doubletrack that climbs a mile up to Mott Peak Trail, everyone's favorite downhill. That would land you back on Abrigo Valley Trail and add almost 2 miles to the overall distance.

After the Ride

Much as Briones is the wildlife staple for many residents of Lafayette–Moraga–Orinda triune (affectionately known to the locals as "Lamorinda"), so is a little restaurant named Chow a staple for the dine-out crowd. A sister restaurant to Park Chow in San Francisco, Chow offers food, yes: a great, eclectic menu; but, more importantly, they feature Death and Taxes on tap—one of the best beers on the planet, brewed in the North Bay by Moonlight Brewery. Even better, this restaurant is located just on the south side of CA 4; take Happy Valley Road from the park back over the hill into town, pass under the highway, and make your first left onto Mount Diablo Boulevard. Then make your third right onto Lafayette Circle, and the restaurant is right there at 53 Lafayette Circle. Call (925) 962-2469 for more information.

05

KEY AT-A-GLANCE INFORMATION

Length: 8.32 miles

Configuration: Clockwise loop

Difficulty: 6/10; very, very steep, but not very technical

Scenery: You can see Mount Diablo in all its glory by looking east across Danville from the ridge top

Exposure: Medium-well. The climb up is the most exposed section of the ride, so consequentially you'll be spending a good amount of time in the sun.

Ride traffic: Low. The severity of the terrain deters the less adventurous.

Riding time: 2–3 hours

Access: Free parking in residential area of Camille Avenue

Facilities: None. Bring a lot of water and sunscreen for this ride.

GPS TRAILHEAD COORDINATES (WGS 84)

UTM Zone 10S
Easting 0585810
Northing 4187660
Latitude N 37° 50' 3.1"
Longitude W 122° 1' 29.2"

LAS TRAMPAS REGIONAL PARK: DEL AMIGO DROP

In Brief

Named after the descent that comes three-fourths of a way through, this ride proves that no matter how jaded you are—despite having ridden everything under the sun—you can still get an adrenaline rush from descending a sixty-story wall such as Del Amigo Trail. Roller coasters have nothing on this descent, and the great part about it is that you actually get to enjoy your time at the top with views across the valley to the majestic Mount Diablo.

DIRECTIONS

By car: From San Francisco, head east across the Bay Bridge on Interstate 80. Once across the bridge, take the Interstate 580 East exit toward Downtown Oakland/Hayward-Stockton/CA 24 and immediately take the CA 24/Grover Shafter Freeway East exit toward Walnut Creek. Drive just over 13 miles to where CA 24 terminates at Interstate 680. Take the I-680 South exit toward San Jose, drive 4.2 miles, and exit onto Stone Valley Road, turning right. From Stone Valley Road, make a left onto Danville Boulevard, drive just over a mile, and then make a right onto Camille Avenue. Drive up Camille to where it dead-ends, and you will see the trailhead sign on the left.

By public transportation: Take the Pittsburg/Bay Point BART train east toward Pittsburg/Bay Point and get off at the Walnut Creek stop. From there, ride south from the BART station on North California Boulevard until you come to the second stoplight (Mount Diablo Boulevard). Make a left onto Mount Diablo Boulevard, ride to South Broadway Boulevard, and make a right. Ride approximately 2 miles down South Broadway Boulevard to where it passes under I-680. From there make a left onto Danville Boulevard, which you'll ride for 2 miles before turning right onto Camille Avenue. Make the first left off Camille Avenue onto Iron Horse Regional Trail and begin the ride.

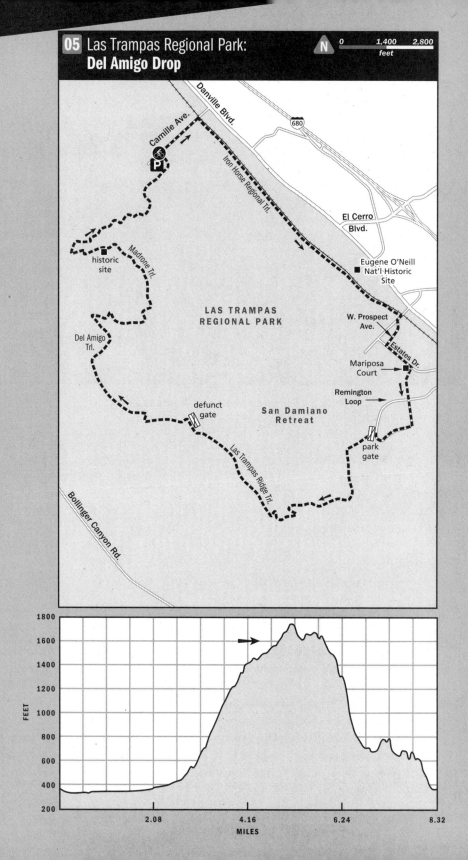

N

0   1,400   2,800
feet

Danville Blvd.

Camille Ave.

P

680

Iron Horse Regional Trl.

El Cerro
Blvd.

historic
site

Madrone Trl.

Eugene O'Neill
Nat'l Historic
Site

LAS TRAMPAS
REGIONAL PARK

Del Amigo
Trl.

W. Prospect
Ave.

Estates Dr.

Mariposa
Court

Remington
Loop

defunct
gate

San Damiano
Retreat

park
gate

Las Trampas Ridge Trl.

Bollinger Canyon Rd

FEET

1800

1600

1400

1200

1000

800

600

400

200

2.08   4.16   6.24   8.32

MILES

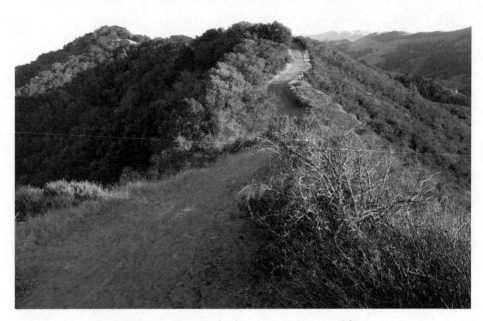

Evening view south along Las Trampas Ridge

Contact

Las Trampas Regional Wilderness
18012 Bollinger Canyon Road
San Ramon, CA 94583
(510) 544-3276
www.ebparks.org/parks/las_trampas

Description

Once you've made the right turn onto Camille Avenue, drive two blocks and park wherever you find space on the street, which is generally not a problem in this quiet neighborhood. Iron Horse Regional Trail is the first left-hand turn from Danville Boulevard and looks like a one-lane road. Ride back to Iron Horse Trail and make a right.

The trail system in the Las Trampas Regional Wilderness doesn't afford mountain bikers with (m)any options for creating loops. They come agonizingly close to affording us one great loop, except for the fact that a simple half-mile section of bike-accessible trail leading from Bollinger Canyon Road to Las Trampas Ridge Trail is missing. That said, this ride incorporates 1.9 miles of the paved, multiuse Iron Horse Trail for the simple facts that a) your legs need a warm up before climbing up onto the ridge, and b) no sensible person would backtrack over Del Amigo Trail just to avoid pavement. Also, Iron Horse Regional Trail is an important experiment for the Bay Area's cycling community and city planners in creating a separate road system for bikes, away from cars. You can read more about this project at **www.ebparks.org/parks/trails/iron_horse.**

Iron Horse Trail intersects five neighborhood streets; on the sixth intersection, make a right onto West Prospect Avenue. Ride three blocks and turn left onto Estates Drive. Ride another three blocks and turn right onto Mariposa Court (which isn't really a court) and then make a right onto Sheri Lane. Ride two blocks up Sheri Lane and make a right onto Remington Drive; proceed straight at the next intersection onto Remington Loop and look for the trailhead on the right, at the base of a medium-size pine tree. Finally, it's trail time. Mark your GPS here, because it should be reading about 440-feet elevation, and in another 2.5 miles you will have climbed all the way up to 1,700 feet.

Remington Loop Trail cuts between two homes and runs along some backyard fences on a southwest bearing for the first 200 yards, climbing easily. The climb gradually steepens as the trail curves left and away from the homes, passing through a cluster of oak trees. Out of the trees the trail makes a right and hits the first intersection.

Head straight through the unmarked intersection, which is where many of the local feeder trails link up with Remington Loop Trail, and click it down a gear or two because this is where the steep starts. In spring, you often see wildflowers scattered on this wide open grassy hillside, if the cattle haven't grazed them first. The trail surface is well maintained, often showing only signs of hoof prints and mild ruts, but even so, with the gradient such as it is, tires with less aggressive tread patterns or overinflated tires will give difficulty with traction.

Coming up on the lip of the ridge, the terrain becomes too steep for even the trail, which starts slithering back onto itself, twisting this way and that so as to avoid cresting. Eventually you reach the top with legs burnings and lungs imploding, and when the torrent of sweat subsides and you regain sight, you might want to turn around and have a look at the view you just earned for yourself. The city of Danville lies on the valley floor, cut in two by the interstate, and beyond that you see the foothills and the great Diablo. Here the trail Ts into Las Trampas Ridge Trail; left takes you down onto private property, while you go right, through the defunct gate, and continue to climb.

The climbing is not quite over. There are approximately 600 more feet to gain in elevation, but these climbs are much more gradual, following the bald top of the ridge. For the next mile and a half, stay on Las Trampas Ridge Trail, which doesn't deviate from the ridgetop, so avoid taking any trails that head down either side of the hill. At mile 5, 1,694 feet elevation, come to a defunct gate and excellent views, particularly to the east, looking past the scraggly old finger of a couple of dead buckeye trees that seem to be reaching out to Mount Diablo in the far off distance. The trail climbs for just another 55 yards past this point to the actual peak at over 1,700 feet elevation, but that section of trail is one of the few bits that is immersed in trees, so you may opt to celebrate the milestone here, y'know, with the sights.

Up and over the nondescript peak begins the downhill portion of the ride. For the next half mile, coast along the spine of the ridge, surrounded by chaparral, and then come to the next major junction. At mile 5.6 make a right onto Del Amigo Trail.

Del Amigo Trail begins innocently enough, curving left and descending lightly to the next intersection with Sulfur Springs Trail. Make a right to stay on Del Amigo Trail and then prepare for the Drop.

After going around a wide right-hand switchback, the trail points itself straight down through the trees. Now, before you get started on this decent (Wily Coyote hangs in the air), be aware that because this trail is so steep and fast, it is easy to get into uncontrollable situations, and this can present a danger both to yourself and other trail users. If you're riding in a group, pull straws to see who gets to be the DD (designated descender) and scout out the trail for the rest of the crew, using a cell phone to call from the bottom and advise on the amount of traffic on the section of trail in question. Otherwise, just exercise extreme caution. Ok, go! SHooSH!!

If you manage to execute the steep off-camber switchbacks coming at the end of 220-yard, 20 percent gradient straightaways, then you find yourself at the bottom of the hill, and it probably only took one or two minutes. That is the Del Amigo Drop. At the bottom you'll see a self-closing ranger gate on the left leading to Madrone Trail. Go through the gate and ride through the cow pasture in the general direction of the buildings at the far end.

To continue with the ride, make your way to the left of the buildings to regain the trail at another gate. Or, if you're a friend of literature and theatre, you may want to call ahead to the Eugene O'Neill National Historic Site (phone (925) 838-0249) and make reservations for a tour of the premises, in which case you can skirt to the right of the ranch house and stroll like mad, sober Hickey down to the large and beautiful Tao House just beyond.

Beyond the pasture, Madrone Trail continues, and this is the most technically interesting section of the ride, but still nowhere near the technical nature of, say, Rockville. Still a fire road, the trail rolls along, occasionally dropping off steeply, all the while winding through the trees and following the crevice in the hill. At the next intersection at mile 7.7, make a right turn, go through the gate, and follow the last bit of trail as it picks a path through the backyards and deposits you back on Camille Avenue.

After the Ride

Probably the best and most reasonably priced private restaurant in Danville is Ha's Restaurant. The food (particularly the curry chicken) is great, and it's right down the street from Las Trampas Regional Park. From Camille, make a right onto Danville Boulevard and drive south until it turns into Hartz Avenue just past Diablo Road. Ha's will be on your left at 531 Hartz Avenue (phone (925) 838-3233).

06

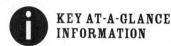

KEY AT-A-GLANCE INFORMATION

Length: 12.13 miles

Configuration: Dog bone

Difficulty: 7/10. Not a challenging ride from a technical standpoint, but the 2,000+ feet of climbing give this ride chutzpah.

Scenery: The view from Antler Point is unbeatable.

Exposure: Burnt—not a whole lotta trees on this ride

Ride traffic: Medium; not a big after-work destination due to the long drive, but popular on weekends

Riding time: 2–3.5 hours

Access: Free parking at the small Grant Lake parking lot

Facilities: Nicer restrooms and water across Mount Hamilton Road at park headquarters

GPS TRAILHEAD COORDINATES (WGS 84)

UTM Zone 10S
Easting 0613810
Northing 4133410
Latitude N 37° 20' 33.3"
Longitude W 121° 42' 58.1"

JOSEPH D. GRANT RANCH COUNTY PARK: EAST LOOPS WITH ANTLER POINT

In Brief

There is a good deal of history behind the 9,553 acres that make up the Joseph D. Grant Ranch County Park, more commonly known as Grant Ranch Park. What does it all add up to? It adds up to one heck of a place to ride, that's what. This dog bone–shaped loop hits all but one of the mountain bike legal trails in the eastern half of the park, also paying a special visit to the Antler Point lookout spot.

Contact

Joseph D. Grant Ranch County Park
18405 Mount Hamilton Road
San Jose, CA 95140
(408) 274-6121
www.sccgov.org/portal/site/parks

Description

Mount Hamilton sits above the south bay like a happy Buddha, offering up a few great leisurely activities. Whether you're in the mood for a simple mountain drive, a visit to the Lick Observatory, or mountain biking at Grant Ranch Park, this is a great place to go to escape

DIRECTIONS

From San Francisco, drive 50 miles south on US 101 to San Jose. On the southern side of San Jose, take the Santa Clara Street/CA 130 exit east (left) toward Alum Rock Avenue. Drive 3.6 miles on Alum Rock Avenue, turn right onto Mount Hamilton Road/CA 130, and drive up the hill, taking care on the narrow roads to watch for road cyclists and other motorists. After about 7.8 miles, you see the main entrance to Joseph D. Grant Ranch County Park on the right, and about 45 yards beyond that, on the left, is the smaller, free Grant Lake parking lot.

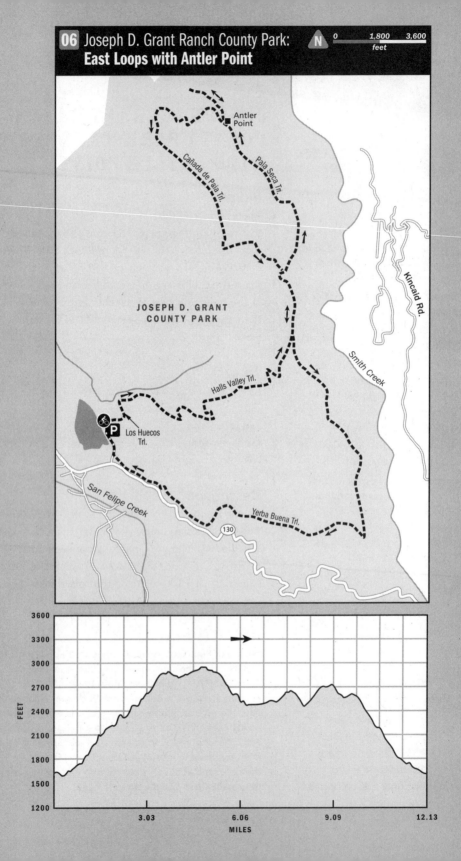

N

0   1,800   3,600
feet

Antler
Point

Cañada de Pala Trl.

Pala Seca Trl.

Kincaid Rd.

Smith Creek

JOSEPH D. GRANT
COUNTY PARK

Halls Valley Trl.

P

Los Huecos
Trl.

San Felipe Creek

Yerba Buena Trl.

130

FEET

3600
3300
3000
2700
2400
2100
1800
1500
1200

3.03   6.06   9.09   12.13
MILES

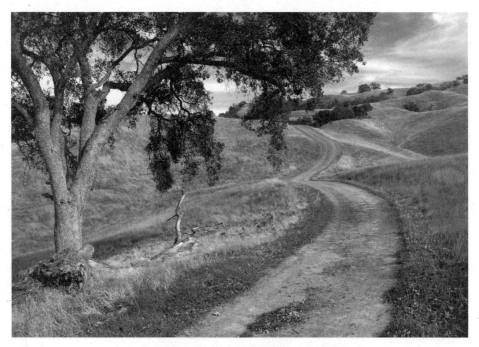

Halls Valley Trail bounds off into the hills.

Silicon Valley, and with the added option of camping at Grant Ranch (for reservations, call (408) 355-2201), your next three-day weekend could very well be spoken for.

For a quick afternoon ride, avoid the $6 parking fee in the main parking lot and drive on another 40 yards (in the uphill direction) to the small Grant Lake parking lot on the left. The trail forks right out of the parking lot. Head right as the left option just leads to a small picnicking area. Ride past the often putrid-smelling Grant Lake to about the midway point and find the intersection with Los Huecos Trail, which is well marked. Turn right onto Los Huecos Trail and ride about 200 yards, and then make a left onto Halls Valley Trail.

Halls Valley Trail is only legal for bikes in the uphill direction. It is one of the windier trails in the park, and rather than constantly entertain the risk of riders descending too quickly around the sharp and often blind turns, park officials opted to close the downhill direction to cyclists. This is a good solution to a specific problem, but it would be nice if mountain bikers could receive some sort of compensatory nod in the form of the occasional downhill mountain-bikers-*only* trail, but who knows if that's ever going to be a reality.

Halls Valley Trail is an excellent 2.1-mile fire-road climb, nonetheless, rolling and twisting its way up the hillside. The bottom portion of the trail is surrounded by coyote brush–dominated chaparral and live oaks, and this gives way to a more open, grassy hillside dotted with valley oaks. The trail surfaces throughout the park are primarily smooth and generally well compacted, meaning that you can enjoy the efficiency of running a higher tire pressure and not have it affect your traction. The trail never gets out of sight, with most of the

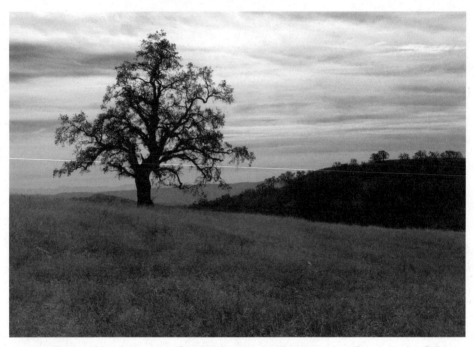

A majestic, old oak, as seen from Pala Seca Trail, appears to dance in the field.

elevation gains making use of drastic switchbacks, which splay the elevation gain out in front of you.

The climb Ts into Cañada de Pala Trail at the top of the ridge, at which point you can check out the views back down to the lake, also noticing the prominent no-bikes sign at the downhill mouth of Halls Valley Trail. Take a left onto Cañada de Pala Trail and ride just under half a mile to the next junction with Pala Seca Trail. Make a right.

Pala Seca Trail keeps climbing along the ridgeline, and by this point, if you're a sea-level dweller, you're probably feeling a bit of the rarified air (okay, so not *that* rarified) in addition to the usual I've-been-climbing-for-almost-4-miles burn in the legs. From the intersection, Pala Seca makes a 7 percent, 440-yard climb and deposits you on the very top of this ridge, leveling out so that you can enjoy the views. To the east you have the motley green mosaic of a tree and chaparral-covered hillside, to the west you have views down to San Jose. This park is renowned for its thriving wildlife, and the last time I was up here, I got to witness two coyotes hunting the grassy hilltop in unison.

When the computer clicks over 4.4 miles, keep an eye open for a little singletrack that peels off on the right, marked with a signpost. This trail doesn't go anywhere, and it's also drastically pitted and roughened up by horses hooves, but it's still a worthwhile excursion, especially if you've got a good suspension setup to smooth things out. The trail takes you up to the top of the peak, to an unassuming little bench presiding over an enormous lookout. There is nothing particularly antler-y about Antler Point itself, probably it was named because it was used by hunters as a spot to sight out the elk that used to roam the hills. Of the 360-degree views, my favorite has to be the views to the south, with the golden undulations of rolling ridgetop surrounded by a sea of green.

Head back down the singletrack and make a right back onto Cañada de Pala Trail, which has wrapped around to meet Pala Seca Trail at this junction. What comes next is a very rapid descent that takes you by the Pala Seca Cabin (aka The Line Shack)—a dilapidated, whitewashed structure that could be seen from Antler Point—all the way down to the floor of Deer Valley. Exercise much care on this descent, as many of the turns are sharp and off-camber—and *steep*: all told, it's a 500-foot drop from Antler Point to the valley floor in just over a mile traveled.

Cañada de Pala Trail rolls through the very picturesque Deer Valley, and the Lick Observatory comes back into view to the distant southeast, although the views of the big white dome are a bit better from the trails in the southern end of the park. The next intersection you come to is with Washburn Trail, on the right. Unfortunately, at the time of writing, the Washburn Trail is misrepresented on the pocket map as being multiuse when actually there is a no-bikes sticker on the signpost and the larger maps posted on the signboards near park headquarters indicate otherwise. Make a left, continuing on Cañada de Pala Trail as it climbs back up to the earlier-encountered intersection with Pala Seca Trail at mile 7.7.

Retrace your tracks past Halls Valley Trail and come to Los Huecos Trail, which you may opt to descend, or you may opt to proceed on another 1.3 miles to Yerba Buena Trail. Both trails offer a very similar get-to-the-bottom experience, but Yerba Buena Trail offers just a bit more bang for your buck. Just a hair shallower than the descent from Antler Point, Yerba Buena Trail runs through 1.3 miles of washboard; sharp, off-camber turns; and loose rocks before hitting Mount Hamilton Road and taking a right to run parallel with the road for a quick-dipping and quarter-mile diving stretch back to the parking lot.

After the Ride

There are a number of taquerias in San Jose, and you might pick Taqueria San Jose simply because it's right on the drive back to the freeway from Grant Ranch—and also because the name sounds so familiar, and if so, your selection would reward you with an inexpensive and highly palatable Mexican eatery. Taqueria San Jose (phone (408) 923-3610) can be found at 235 East Santa Clara Street in San Jose.

07

DIABLO FOOTHILLS: FOOTHILLS TO ALAMO LOOP

ⓘ KEY AT-A-GLANCE INFORMATION

Length: 4.53 miles

Configuration: Clockwise loop with 0.3-mile out-and-back midride to see the Castle Rocks formations

Difficulty: 3/10; on the shorter side, with a couple of steep climbs and a steep, twisty final descent

Scenery: Diablo looms, but the real site here are the strange rock formations found in the southwest corner of the park.

Exposure: Well-done

Ride traffic: High

Riding time: 0.75–1.25 hours

Access: Free parking; park is open later than most, until 10 p.m.

Facilities: None

In Brief

This is a great jaunt in the hills, particularly if you live in the area and prefer the outdoors to a treadmill. The park itself isn't very large, but the fact that it's a gateway to Mount Diablo State Park and Shell Ridge Open Space means it will provide many an evening of exploration.

Contact

Diablo Foothills Regional Park
1700 Castle Rock Road
Walnut Creek, CA 94598
(925) 945-8244
www.ebparks.org/parks/diablo_foothills

DIRECTIONS

By car: From San Francisco, head east across the Bay Bridge on Interstate 80. Once across the bridge, take the Interstate 580 East exit toward downtown Oakland/Hayward-Stockton/CA 24 and immediately take the CA 24/Grover Shafter Freeway East exit toward Walnut Creek. Drive just over 13 miles to where CA 24 terminates at Interstate 680. Take the I-680 S exit toward San Jose, drive 3.3 miles, and take the Livorna Road exit, making a left onto Livorna Road. Drive 1.5 miles up Livorna Road and look for the Livorna Staging Area parking lot on the left. Past this point are gated communities, so you'll know if you've gone too far.

By public transportation: Take the Pittsburg/Bay Point BART train east toward Pittsburg/Bay Point and get off at the Walnut Creek stop. From there, ride south from the BART station on North California Boulevard until you come to the second stoplight, which is Mount Diablo Boulevard. Make a left onto Mount Diablo Boulevard, ride to South Broadway Boulevard, and make a right. Ride approximately 2 miles down South Broadway Boulevard to where it passes under I-680, and from there make a left onto Danville Boulevard, which you'll ride 0.3 miles before turning left onto Livorna Road, passing back under the freeway, and riding a half mile to the parking lot.

GPS TRAILHEAD COORDINATES (WGS 84)

UTM Zone 10S
Easting 0587160
Northing 4191750
Latitude N 37° 52' 15.5"
Longitude W 122° 0' 32.6"

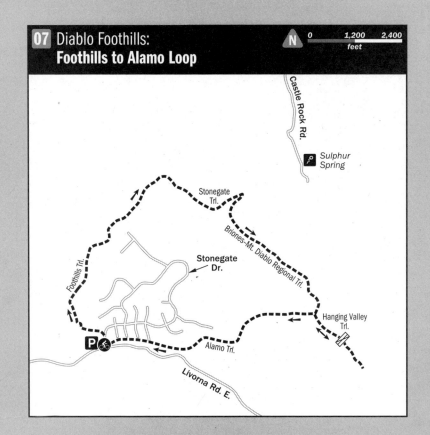

07 Diablo Foothills: Foothills to Alamo Loop

N 0   1,200   2,400
feet

Castle Rock Rd.

Sulphur Spring

Stonegate Trl.

Briones-Mt. Diablo Regional Trl.

Foothills Trl.

Stonegate Dr.

Hanging Valley Trl.

P

Alamo Trl.

Livorna Rd. E.

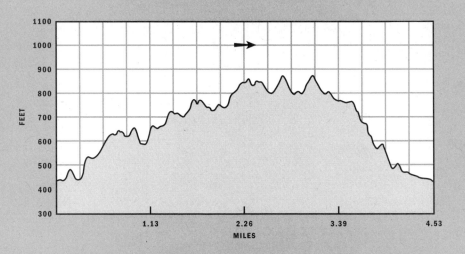

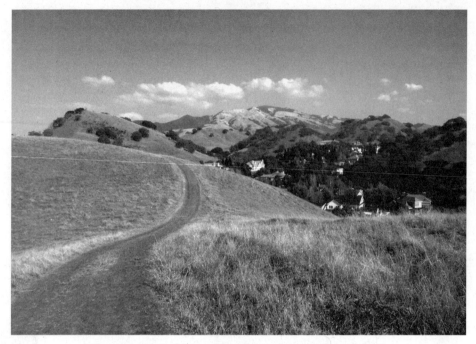

Foothills Trail climbs above the nearby neighborhood.

Description

Once known as "Nuts Creek," Walnut Creek is a well-to-do city located 24 miles northeast of San Francisco where CA 24 hits the base of Mount Diablo. The city is known for having a high ratio of open space to people, and that, combined with the ease of public transportation into the city, means that this city is popular with San Francisco professionals who want to settle with families outside of the hustle and bustle.

The trailheads at the Livorna Staging Area are somewhat obscure, hidden among the guarded gates and high fences of the wealthy communities that this ride circuits. Locate the trailhead signboard at the east end of the lot; here you can pick up a trail map. Foothills Trail continues right, past the signboard, following a tiny swath of open space set aside just for it. A manicured, pea-graveled doubletrack slips between a few of the estates and out into the grassy open and immediately, magically turns into singletrack.

Just past the backyard fences, the trail attempts to flee the coop, climbing steeply onto the ridge. The climb is not sustained, though, and a descent follows soon after, running past a small pond, before resuming the climb up the foothills.

The first intersection, with Hazard Hill Trail, comes quickly; make a right to stay on Foothills Trail. Hazard Hill Trail is the first option out of Diablo Foothills Regional Park and into Shell Ridge Open Space, which is but one of the great options for extending this ride. Here the trail turns into fire road. Click it into low gear, because the climbing starts again. A second intersection with Hazard Hill comes just 65 yards later; stay to the right on Foothills Trail.

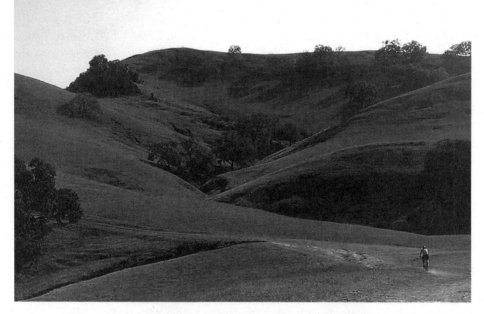

**A rider rides down Briones–Mount Diablo Trail
in the direction of the Castle Rock formations.**

By now you've ascended above the surrounding homes, and you can start to see down into some of the landscaped backyards in addition to the views up to the Devil itself. The trail rolls through the first mile, then hits another quick descent, bringing you into an area of confusing trail junctures. One of frustrating things about this park is the almost complete lack of trail markers.

At mile 1.3, make a soft right onto Twin Ponds Trail, which passes through an old barbed-wire fence, climbing slightly. In the next 110 yards, make two left turns at unmarked intersections, ignoring the water tank access trail and the continuation of Foothills Trail, respectively. About 0.2 miles later, come to another four-way junction and make a 90-degree left turn onto Stonegate Trail, which ramps up the grade to 7 percent, aiming for the valley between two mild peaks. At the top of this small climb, you come to yet another four-way intersection, where Stonegate Trail Ts into Briones–Mount Diablo Regional Trail. Buckeye Ravine Trail continues out the back, but that's restricted to hiker use only.

Make the sharp right turn onto Briones–Mount Diablo Regional Trail, which levels out, passing over a mild rocky section and cuts to the left of a small pond. The pond is often dry in late summer, which makes the hieroglyphic NO SWIMMING sign somewhat comical. The trail follows a small stream up the hill, at the top of which the stream disappears underground and Mount Diablo comes into full view. The site line to the top is almost completely unobstructed, with just a few distant homes dotting the hillside and the cell tower at the top.

Oak trees are scattered everywhere, and in late fall the yellow grassy hills are dotted with the fading green of the oak trees, which cast orange shadows of discarded leaves. Also from here, looking west, away from Mount Diablo, you'll catch a glimpse of a very strange rock outcropping sitting on a small rise, looking very much like the Rock Biter character from the movie *The Neverending Story*. You can't just let a sight like that go unexplored, now can you? No, it's time for a little detour.

At the bottom of a quick descent, Hanging Valley splits off to the right. In order to complete the loop, you will be taking Hanging Valley Trail, but for the moment, make the left at this intersection, staying on Briones–Mount Diablo Trail. The trail flattens out, heading toward a gigantic old oak, but don't be too enchanted by the tree, because there is a washout slowly eating away at the left-hand side of the trail, three feet across at points, and when the lighting is just right (well, wrong), this can be almost invisible until the last second. If you're carrying your speed from the descent, just be sure to err to the right.

Beyond the washout, the trail climbs another 220 yards up to a gate defining the boundary of Mount Diablo State Park. Pass through the gate, and as you head down the fire road, the amazing rock formations come into view. This particular formation is known as the China Wall, earning that title because of how the sandstone has pushed up through the soil to form a long, surprisingly straight wall of varying height. There are other rock formations to be found throughout the open space, notably the Castle Rock formations, which could be another good diversion to add some length to this ride (see the Diablo Foothills Regional Park map to get an idea of what trails to take to get to the Castle Rock Recreation Area). When you've finished admiring the rocks, turn around and ride back up to the gate.

Back at the intersection with Hanging Valley Trail, make a left and head 0.3 miles down the hill to the next junction. Here, make a left onto Alamo Trail. (If you're interested in seeing more rock formations, you can take a right onto Hanging Valley Trail and ride just 220 yards to where the trail passes by another, smaller set of natural rock walls.)

Alamo Trail is a surprisingly, for this park, steep and technical singletrack descent through a dense young oak forest. There is only one other intersection to be concerned with at this point. When you reach it, make a right. The descent lands you on a gravel multiuse path that passes behind a row of backyard fences and takes you back out to Livorna Road.

After the Ride

For a post-ride pasta fix, get back on I-680 and head toward CA 24, but detour to Salvatore Italian Restaurant at 1627 North Broadway in Walnut Creek. Exit Rudgear Road off I-680 and turn right onto Rudgear Road. Then immediately turn left onto South Broadway. Drive just over a mile to where South Broadway turns into North Broadway, and the restaurant will be on your left. With creative appetizers and an excellent bar, this smallish mom-and-pop is not your average Italian chain restaurant (phone (925) 932-2828).

08

KEY AT-A-GLANCE INFORMATION

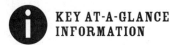

Length: 8.1 miles

Configuration: Dog bone

Difficulty: 7/10; difficulty attributed to steepness and length

Scenery: South Bay vistas, beautiful Mission Peak itself

Exposure: Well-done. You'll sweat, so bring a small bottle of sunscreen with you.

Ride traffic: Moderate; hikers and hang gliders on Hidden Valley Loop

Riding time: 2.25–3 hours

Access: Free parking in lot

Facilities: Restrooms and water fountains

GPS TRAILHEAD COORDINATES (WGS 84)

UTM Zone 10S
Easting 0596620
Northing 4151170
Latitude N 37° 30' 15.7"
Longitude W 121° 54' 25.3"

MISSION PEAK: MISSION PEAK LOOP

In Brief

Climbing up to Mission Peak is no cakewalk, but just like going to the moon, a lot of energy output results in a cool view of Earth. From the austere, windswept vantage point atop the peak, to the hang gliders circling the base, this ride has a lot of aspects that set it apart from other rides, and that allows you to overlook the relatively mundane quality of the trail itself. Coming back down the wide, smooth fire roads will have you feeling like a 1990s-era John Tomac racing down Mammoth Mountain.

Contact

Mission Peak Regional Preserve
East end of Stanford Avenue, off Mission Boulevard
Fremont, CA 94538
(925) 862-2244
www.ebparks.org/parks/mission

Description

Looking up at Mission Peak from the Stanford Avenue parking lot, you can see pretty much all of what the day

DIRECTIONS

By car: From San Francisco, drive approximately 17 miles south on US 101 to CA 92. Exit CA 92 east toward Hayward and cross over the bay. After 13 miles exit onto Interstate 880 South toward San Jose. Take the Warren Avenue/Mission Boulevard exit, merging onto Mission Boulevard. Turn left on Stanford Avenue and drive 1 mile up the hill to the parking lot.

By public transportation/bike: Take the Fremont-bound BART to the last stop in Fremont. From the station, take a left onto Civic Center Drive, a right onto Walnut Avenue, and then another left onto Paseo Padre Parkway. Paseo Padre Parkway is a bike-friendly street: ride it for approximately 5.5 miles and then make a left onto South Grimmer Boulevard. Make a right onto Mission Boulevard and then a left onto Stanford Avenue.

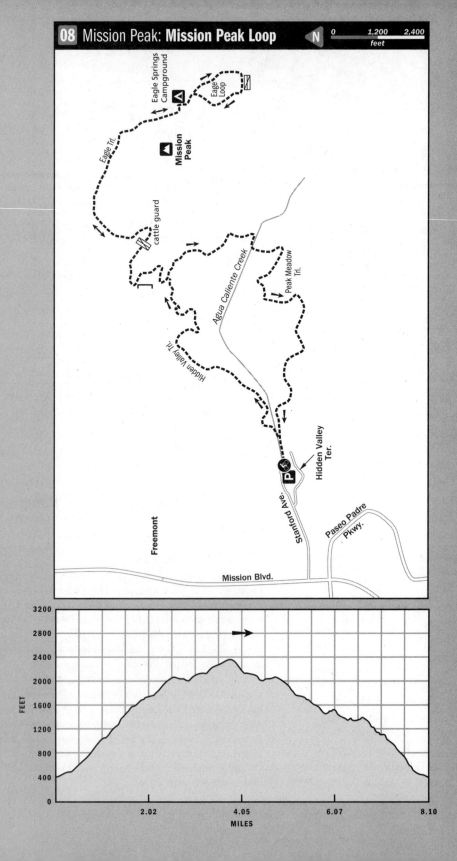

has in store for you. The geography of the mountain face is not very complex, and the high exposure leaves much of the steep fire-road trails visible to you. But don't let yourself be deterred! Just click it in a low gear, go through the gate, and start spinning.

At the first fork, make a left onto Hidden Valley Trail, which is where the climbing starts. The tendency of hikers to use this more direct route up the hill is the reason why this loop is best in a clockwise fashion. This gives you the opportunity, on the way down Peak Meadow Trail, to be a little freer with your speed.

The lower portion of Hidden Valley Trail is a ridiculously well-maintained gravel fire road. If you hit the park in the afternoon, chances are good that you will see some of the many hang gliders that make use of the park's steep slopes and predictable wind patterns to enjoy their sport. Hidden Valley Trail runs right through one of their favorite landing zones. Watch your head.

I won't lie to you: the trails in this park are steep! There are some very good switchback turns heading up Hidden Valley Trail, but despite the effort of builders to relax the gradient, it's still a rough one to climb. You must be a climb-loving masochist to truly love this park, I think, or just have faith or knowledge that the views from the top are going to be well worth it (they are). Another good reason for climbing rather than descending Hidden Valley Trail is the fact that there are a couple well-placed shady spots along this way. Peak Meadow Trail is devoid of these nice little rest areas, and so climbing that trail, though just as steep, is made more difficult by the exposure.

As you head up Hidden Valley Trail, be sure to take in the views of the lower slopes, which are patterned with interesting, tight concentric circles looking very much like topography marks from a map. These lines are actually trails carved into the hillsides by the cattle that graze through there. It's a pretty sight.

At mile 1.5 turn left at the fork. Note that the trail that splits off here is Peak Meadow Trail, which you'll turn onto on your descent. There is more—how do you say—steep climbing to be had here. On the plus side, the views are really starting to open up! And as you fall over gasping for air again, maybe take a look behind you and catch some of the hang gliders taking off below.

Another quarter mile nets you a bench for your suffering, where you might want to stop and enjoy the view if you haven't already. Just 55 yards past this is a beautiful rock outcropping with strange red moss on it, and this is mirrored by the rock and red moss on the face of Mission Peak just behind it.

The familiar chatter of spoked wheels on cattle guards announces your arrival at the base of Mission Peak's face. The hillsides open up into a small meadow at the base of the peak. There is an abundance of ground squirrels here, all running around and playing. Turn left at the next fork, mile 2.2, continuing on Hidden Valley Trail. The right option is Grove Trail, which leads across the face of Mission Peak to an in-park residence.

Continue right at the next fork on Hidden Valley Trail. A barbed-wire fence runs down and terminates at this point. It doesn't contain anything, which is strange. At the end of the barbed-wire fence are two wooden sections, which look like they must have once been the two sides of a now nonexistent gate. Climb through the opening made by these two things. The whole deal is really very Cristo—a fence that does nothing. Notice the rocky patch here

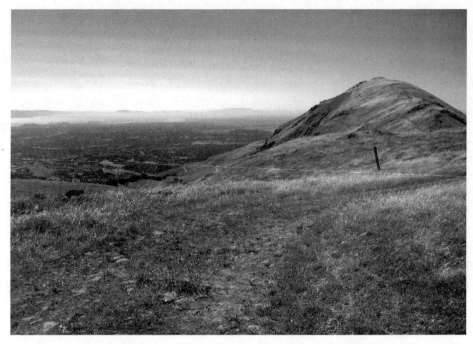

The South Bay, as seen from the shoulder of Mission Peak

as you climb up through the old gate opening; you'll be descending back over this section in a bit, so just take note of it. From here the trail devolves into rough doubletrack, maintained only by tires of the forest service vehicles that pass through. The trail is considerably rockier through here.

Cresting over the ridge, you wind up on the backside of the peak to the north. The whole area is open to cattle. There are incredible views from here. The backside of the peak is almost wholly undeveloped, and the yellow grassy hills roll off into the distance. When you come to the next fork, you'll make a left. If you happened to bring a lock, you could lock your bike to one of the signposts and walk up the trail that runs over the top of the peak.

Turn right onto Eagle Trail at the next fork, and in about another 20 yards, you come onto the Eagle Springs Backpack Camp. There is a hand-pump water spigot here if you need to fill up. Continue heading right, past the camp and up the hill on the doubletrack. The views from the backside of the peak are amazing as they are almost totally unadulterated.

A few yards up the hill from the camp, there is a trail signpost, but the trail it points to is virtually nonexistent. Presumably it was once a fire road like all of the other trails in the park, but time and lack of use have seen it overgrown with grass. Most people, particularly those on foot, choose to go right at this intersection and double-back once they've caught the view. But, as a mountain biker, we have an instinct and a desire for loops, and if given the option to do a loop, by golly we'll do a loop! So go left at this signpost and keep a keen eye out for the trail. It almost resembles a singletrack, so you should be happy, as it will be the closest to that you're going to get on this ride. Just keep in mind that the trail more or less follows the barbed-wire fence running along there; as long as you keep that fence to your left, you're on the right track. Climb up this trail, knowing full well that you are doing your part to resurrect it back to its former glory. When the fence turns right, you turn right.

The trail runs across another gate, which leads to the south. This is the access point to Monument Peak, which is another 4 miles or so off in the distance beyond the cell towers you'll see there. Don't pass through the gate, stay on Eagle Loop. Another 30 feet on and *voila!* The ridge drops away and you are slapped with some incredible views of the South Bay Area. Mission Peak lies just to your right, and you are almost on a level with it. From here there are incredible views of Fremont, Union City, and the patterned and colorful South Bay watershed. The wind will likely be whipping in your face, so it's not the greatest place to stop for a snack, but do take a moment to enjoy this visual you've worked so hard for.

Continue on Eagle Loop, and you'll come to the well-worn portion. Make a right at the fork, as left is the hiking-only trail seen from the other side that passes directly over the summit. Head back down to Eagle Springs Backpack Camp, and then you will backtrack for the next 1.8 miles to the intersection of Hidden Valley and Peak Meadow trails and turn left onto the latter trail.

Peak Meadow Trail rolls along the hillside at the base of Mission Peak. It is rolling terrain for the first 0.75 miles, and there are some great shady spots as it rolls through a surprisingly lush live-oak and bay forest, which is fed by the small McClure Spring. Looking up and down the hill at the green swath cutting through the dry, grassy hillside gives an idea of the power of a little bit of water in an ecosystem such as this. This trail is frequented by equestrians, and some of the turns are blind, so be sure to take it easy on the gas.

After exiting the woods, the trail climbs for a few hundred yards before coming to a fork. There is a small, usually dry pond and the skeleton of an old dead oak tree nestled inside the turn. Beyond that a rock outcropping that sits on the precipice of the ridge overlooks the city below. It's a picturesque spot reminiscent of old Western films. Go right at the fork and continue down Peak Meadow Trail. This is a steep, roaring downhill, and the trail is mostly visible from top to bottom. Scanning ahead for traffic will inform your speed potential. Toward the bottom the trail enters a eucalyptus stand, passes through a gate and over a bridge, and then winds up back at the junction with Hidden Valley Trail. Just keep heading downhill, and you'll wind up back at the parking lot. Your weary legs will thank you.

This is a brutally steep ride, and unless you're a psycho climber type, you'll probably only do this ride once. The views really are stunning, though, and the view from the outermost point of Eagle Loop is as good as it gets.

After the Ride

Head over to the Tia Juana Bar & Grill at 3839 Washington Boulevard (phone (510) 659-8036). Just take Paseo Padre Boulevard north about 3 miles to Washington Boulevard, make a left, and then drive another 1.5 miles on Washington Boulevard. It's in a strange location, but the food and service at this place are top-notch.

Length: 8.76 miles

Configuration: Counterclockwise loop

Difficulty: 7/10; leg-snapping steep

Scenery: 2,300-foot sightlines, oak and Coulter pine forest, chaparral, and thriving fauna

Exposure: Well-done. Top of the climb is most exposed, and that's where you'll naturally be spending the most time.

Ride traffic: Weekdays, mild; weekends and holidays, high

Riding time: 2–2.75 hours

Access: $3 parking fee, open 8 a.m. to sunset

Facilities: Nice restrooms and water fountains at trailhead, also a ranger office where you can buy large maps and get info on trail conditions

GPS TRAILHEAD COORDINATES (WGS 84)

UTM Zone 10S
Easting 0593080
Northing 4197260
Latitude N 37° 55' 12"
Longitude W 121° 56' 27.5"

MOUNT DIABLO STATE PARK: EAGLE PEAK LOOP

In Brief

If the climbs featured in the rest of the East Bay rides just haven't been steep enough and long enough for you, then you should really consider a trip to good old Mount Diablo, the tallest park in this region known for its leg-crushingly steep climbs. This ride attacks the north side of the mountain, circumnavigating Eagle Peak, one of the minor players at a full 1,500 feet lower elevation than the Mount Diablo Summit, via Mitchell Canyon Fire Road.

Contact

Mount Diablo State Park
96 Mitchell Canyon Road
Clayton CA 94517
(925) 837-2525
www.parks.ca.gov/?page_id=517

Description

First thing you see when driving into the Mitchell Canyon Park headquarters and staging area is a mining operation on your right, exhibiting gigantic gray terraces carved into the faces of two nearby adjoining hills. Remember these geological perversions, as they will serve

DIRECTIONS

From San Francisco, head east across the Bay Bridge on Interstate 80. Once across the bridge, take the Interstate 580 East exit toward downtown Oakland/Hayward-Stockton/CA 24 and immediately take the CA 24/Grover Shafter Freeway East exit toward Walnut Creek. Drive just over 13 miles to where CA 24 terminates at Interstate 680. Take the I-680 North exit toward Concord/Sacramento, keep right, and in just under a mile, exit onto Ygnacio Valley Road. Drive 7.5 miles up Ygnacio Valley Road and turn right on Clayton Road. Drive another mile and turn right onto Mitchell Canyon Road, which will take you right up to park headquarters.

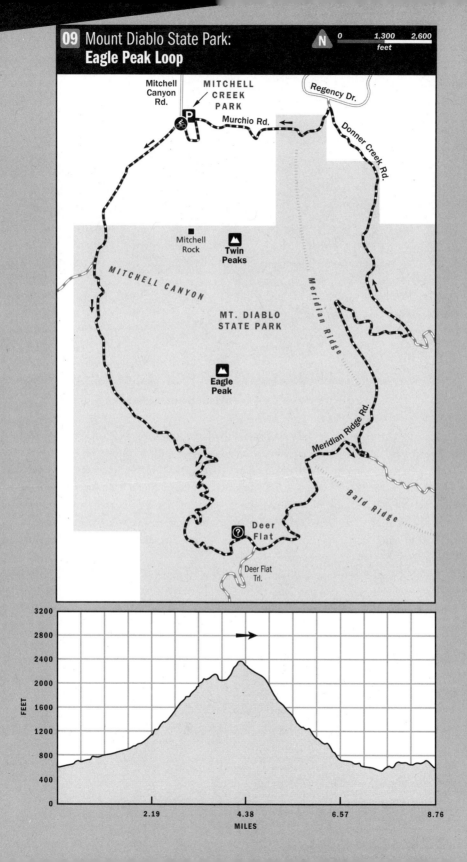

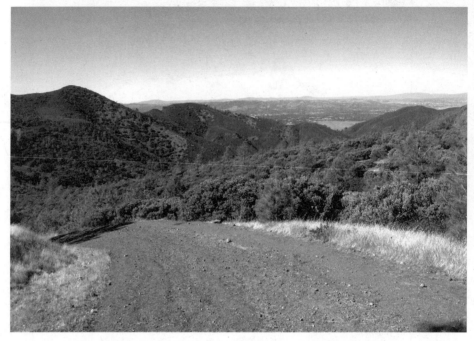

Looking back down the (steep) climb up to Meridian Ridge

as important landmarks later on in the ride. Fifty-five yards from the actual parking lot there is an awkward self-serve parking meter placed in the middle of the narrow two-lane road. Parking fee is $3 and requires that you fill out your vehicle info on a tiny envelope and stuff it in a slot that's difficult to reach from most car windows. It's a little inconvenient, especially when there are a few people driving in at once, but hey, it's a park. It's not supposed to work as efficiently as the Bay Bridge toll plaza, right? Once inside, you enter the large gravel parking lot ringed by large black oaks, which, during fall, drop fantastically large acorns a-thump on the roofs of parked cars.

With a starting elevation of 600 feet, Mitchell Canyon fire road takes off, innocently enough, from a ranger gate at the north end of the parking lot. The trail is very well maintained, climbing slightly up through a canopy of expressive young oak trees that soon begin to intermix with Coulter pines and eventually more chaparral-esque plant life as you work your way up the hill. You should always wear a helmet when riding, but it becomes especially poignant when the humungous pinecones from the Coulter pines are dropping in fall. These prickly beasts can pack a wallop!

Ignore all intersection trails for the first 3.5 miles, as you'll be taking Mitchell Canyon fire road all the way up, following Mitchell Creek, to Deer Flat. Most intersecting trails are singletracks, anyhow, and it's a good rule of thumb to remember that mountain bikes are allowed on none of the singletracks in and around Mount Diablo (this includes Diablo Foothills Regional Park and Morgan Territory). This is a very pretty climb with the creek feeding the greenery. There is a vibrant culture of wild grape vines running throughout, and in the fall, the large leaves put off a bright red color to rival the best any poison oak's got. The canyon is protected from all but the most well-aimed northern wind, and listening to the powerful winds ripping from west to east across the tops of the ridges is a nice counterpoint to your own heavy breathing, which you'll notice increasing in magnitude as the gradient gets steeper and steeper.

The park is popular with all manner of enthusiasts, and though you may find it easy to outpace your wheelless trail companions on the lower pitches of Mitchell Canyon fire road, you may find it more difficult to hold them off as the pitch turns up, right about the 2.3 mile mark. When the trail cuts left, crossing the creek over a culvert, then the real trouble starts. The gradient ramps up to a fervent 12 percent, and the trail surface begins to exhibit increased rocky texturing. Attempts were made to ease the climb, with numerous switchbacks thrown in, but they do little. If you can ride to the top without stopping, then you belong on the National Mountain Bike Series (NMBS) cross-country or marathon circuit. For those that must put a foot down, at least you're greeted with some amazing views, staring down into the valley past a trailside buckeye or coyote brush.

The twisting, upward onslaught finally relents at mile 3.5, depositing you at Deer Flat, a level spot on top of the ridge and a great spot for a snack. There are benches here, set in among more Coulter pines and black oaks, allowing one to take advantage of the 2,000-foot view while enjoying a snack. An info board at the site has labeled pictures of some of the flora and fauna found on the mountain. Three trails intersect here: Mitchell Canyon Trail, which you rode up on, essentially turns into Meridian Ridge Trail, while Deer Flat Trail peels off to the right. Should you suspect that you'll need more than a 2,400-foot elevation maximum on your ride, then you can make the right on Deer Flat Trail and make your way up toward Mount Diablo Summit and the visitor center there. Unfortunately, there aren't many loops available for mountain bikers around the summit—most of the fire roads are either connected by hiker trails, paved roads, or in some cases they dead-end completely. That said, there is a lot of good riding in the park, and on another day you could head over to Curry Canyon on the south side of the mountain and check out a couple of the great loops there, but for today, ignore Deer Flat Trail and make the left onto Meridian Ridge Trail.

From Deer Flat, the trail descends a bit, crossing Deer Flat Creek, a small stream—dry throughout much of the year—that cuts across the trail but presents few technical challenges beyond deep gravel. From there, though, the trail pitches up for a very steep 660-yard section fraught with loose billiard-ball-size rocks. The rocks aren't as colorful as billiard balls, but the poison oak alongside the trail can be during the fall months.

Where this climb crests, the trail intersects Eagle Peak Trail, which is a great single-track cutting straight over the top of Eagle Peak. Great, that is, if you're a hiker, as this trail is no-bikes, so make a right at this intersection, keeping on Meridian Ridge Trail as it drops off the ridge to the east of Eagle Peak.

This is a great descent with minimal punctuation, the first comma coming approximately 0.4 miles past the Eagle Peak junction, where you make a sharp left at the intersection with Prospector's Gap fire road to stay on Meridian Ridge fire road. There is some serious rock texturing happening on this descent, which will put your suspension and/or arms to good abuse. Rocks are small to large, fixed and loose.

From the left at Prospector's Gap, the trail shoots right down the back of Meridian Ridge and since the ridge is covered in chaparral and not trees, you have just amazing views on all sides, in addition to excellent trail visibility. At the brow of the ridge, the trail makes a sharp right, doubling back to the southeast and descending another 0.4 miles to the intersection with Donner Creek fire road.

Make a left onto Donner Creek fire road and continue down the hill (although Cardinet Road to the right offers a stellar, switchback-filled, out-and-back 2,500-foot climb up to Mount Olympia, if you're interested). As the trail continues to descend to sub-1,000-feet elevations, suddenly the mined mountains seen on the drive into the park come back into view. Keep these landmarks in view, because the trail signage in this area of the park is inexplicably confusing. There are many trail junctions and not nearly enough correct trail signs by which one may get bearings. From here it should be a simple mile through the foothills back to the parking lot, but if you're unfamiliar with the area, that mile can easily turn into 3 confused, lost miles.

Contrary to what is listed on the free handout map that many people wind up with (since most do not want to drop $6 on the full map), you need to take a left on Murchio Road. There *is* a sign marking this trail, although Murchio Road is obscured in a very tiny font while the destination, Water Tower Road, is writ large. In my humble opinion, it would make more sense to foreground the name of the trail one is immediately looking for and then provide a smaller indication of destination (and perhaps a true destination, like Mitchell Canyon Staging Area, not another far-off trail).

So, with Water Tower Road and the mined mountains as your talismans, make your steady way back to Mitchell Canyon Staging Area. You can take either Oak Road (not on any map) or Murchio Road at this point, so long as you're heading in the direction of the mines. Eventually you will ride past the eponymous water tower and wind up on a bluff overlooking the parking lot. There is no direct trail to the parking lot from here; you must head left along the bluff to where Water Tower Road intersects Mitchell Canyon fire road, just a stone's throw away.

After the Ride

The only real destination in Clayton that isn't a part of the city's chain-store explosion is Ed's Mudville Grill. This is a great, upscale sports bar/pub in the center of Old Town Clayton (which is ironically undergoing renovation and revitalization), with a huge menu and great atmosphere. To get there, drive back down Mitchell Canyon Road to Clayton Road, turn right, and drive a quarter mile to Oak Street, turn right, and then make your first left onto Center Street. Ed's Mudville Grill is hard to miss on your left, at 6200 Center Street (phone (925) 673-0333).

10

KEY AT-A-GLANCE INFORMATION

Length: 9.17 miles

Configuration: Clockwise with 0.56-mile out-and-back

Difficulty: 7/10. Steep terrain, but not technical; look out for "the Wall" at the end

Scenery: Many ridgetop views and springtime flowers, but this park is renowned for what is underground.

Exposure: Well-done

Ride traffic: Ease of access for the burgeoning communities off of US 4 means that ride traffic is generally high during the typical leisure hours.

Riding time: 2.5–3.25 hours

Access: $5 parking fee. Park at upper lot, if space is available; otherwise lower lot provides for plenty of overflow parking.

Facilities: Outhouse, drinking fountains, and free maps at the trailhead

GPS TRAILHEAD COORDINATES (WGS 84)
UTM Zone   10S
Easting   0599940
Northing   4201590
Latitude   N 37° 57' 30.4"
Longitude   W 121° 51' 44.4"

BLACK DIAMOND MINES REGIONAL PRESERVE: LARK TRAIL TO THE WALL

In Brief

This park is split in two halves: a western and an eastern half. Since the western half is less desirable, consisting of steeper terrain and less loop-able trail options, this ride makes a large circumference of the more tenable eastern side of the park, starting from the Somersville Townsite and winding up with what is known locally as "the Wall"— a leg-smashing climb that brings you back up and over the ridge from the abandoned Stewartsville Townsite.

Contact

Black Diamond Mines Regional Preserve
5175 Somersville Road
Antioch, CA 94509
(925) 757-2620
www.ebparks.org/parks/black_diamond

Description

The Somersville Townsite was one of five that existed in the area during the coal-mining boom that occurred in

DIRECTIONS

From San Francisco, take Interstate 80 across the Bay Bridge toward Oakland. Once across the bridge, be in the right lane and take the Interstate 580 East exit toward Downtown Oakland/CA 24, drive 1.7 miles, and take the CA 24 East exit toward Walnut Creek. Drive 13 miles on CA 24 and take the Interstate 680 exit north toward Concord/Sacramento. Drive 7.4 miles on I-680 and exit onto CA 4 East toward Antioch/Pittsburg. Drive 13.3 miles and exit at Somersville Road/Auto Center Drive, turn right, and head south on Somersville Road for just over 2 miles. You come to the attendant's booth at the opening of the parking lot for the park offices. Drive another half mile up the road and park at the trailhead in the upper parking lot in the Somersville Townsite.

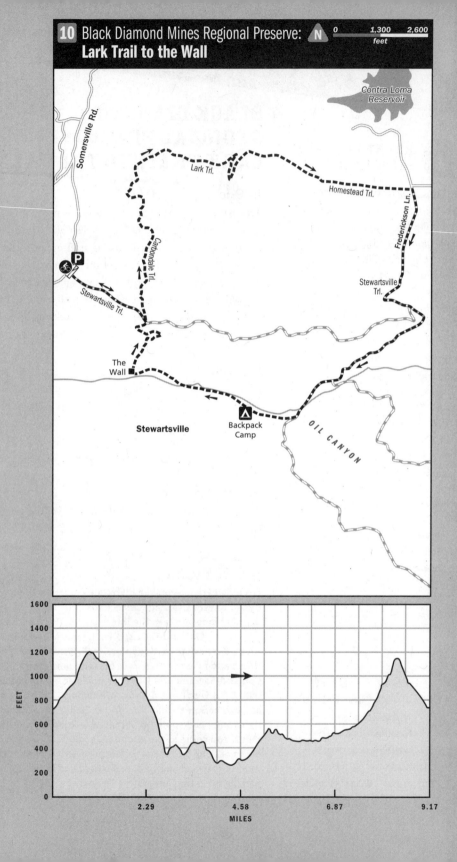

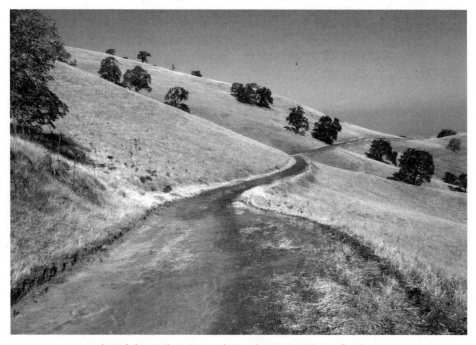

Carbondale Trail passing through a scattering of oak trees

the late 1800s. When the "black diamond" bubble burst, they switched to mining sand, and when the sand ran out, they switched back to the ranching that predated all of the mining. As of today, the preserve comprises almost 6,000 acres, which is accessed by more than 65 miles of trails and fire roads. Maybe, now that the California housing bubble has seemingly burst, the major developments will stay focused around CA 4, and we can hope to enjoy this preserve for another couple hundred years.

Pass through the gate at the far end of the upper parking lot and pedal 75 yards on Nortonville Trail to where you make a left onto Stewartsville Trail. Stewartsville Trail pops over a steep pitch and passes through a gate before meeting Railroad Bed Trail on the left. Continue straight on Stewartsville Trail as it passes through a small grove of nonnative trees that the miners introduced. Just out of the trees, you pass the Pittsburg Mine Trail—well marked as NO-BIKES—and Stewartsville Trail starts climbing in earnest up the grassy, treeless hillside.

The long slog brings you up to the top of the ridge at 1,100 feet and the next intersection, for an elevation gain of over 400 feet in just under a mile from the parking lot. Make a left here onto Carbondale Trail, which runs north and cuts to the right of the nearby peak. From here you can see the long fingers of the bay that provide a backdrop for the towns along CA 4, of which Antioch and Pittsburg are visible from the ridges of this preserve. Unfortunately, a considerable amount of smog collects in this part of the bay area, and it can obscure some of the views.

Just north of the peak, the trail intersects Saddle Trail on the left. If you forgot your water bottles and need to head back to the car, this is a good route; otherwise stay on Carbondale Trail and head down the steep descent. This descent makes a sharp left off the ridge and then swoops into a broad right-hander, passing to the left of a reed-shrouded pond nestled in the base of the contour between hills.

Oak trees dot the hillsides of the park, congregating in the water-rich crevices, but for the most part, the park is open, and the benefit of this is that you can safely scan ahead for traffic and adjust speeds on the downhills to suit. When the fire roads have recently been grated, traction can suffer on the sandy, clump-prone soil base, until the weather and trail users have had time to tamp it down; the slowing effect is true both climbing and descending these hills.

From the pond the trail climbs steadily for a half mile up to the next junction, where you make a right to stay on Carbondale Trail. The descending begins here; just less than 0.2 miles to the right, turn onto Lark Trail, and another 0.5 miles or so down, there is a 14 percent grade to the bottom of the canyon. The cut of this descent is slightly blind, so be ready to stop safely if surprised by other trail users.

At the bottom make a sharp right to stay on Lark Trail and climb 175 yards and make a left onto Homestead Trail, which introduces itself as a mild climb but quickly turns into yet another steep descent. If you carry your speed, you can make it over the two-story hurdle at the bottom on momentum alone, but take it easy, as the approach can be rough, with some ruts and exposed rocks. At the top of the hurdle is the next intersection. Head straight on Homestead Trail, avoiding *Old* Homestead *Loop*, which veers off to the right.

Homestead Trail runs into a parking lot at the northeast corner of the park, which is kitty-corner to the Contra Loma Regional Park. If you're dying from the heat and you've got a couple extra bucks in your pack for beach fees, then you could head over to the Contra Loma lagoon for a swim. If you're in no such need, make a right at the parking lot onto Stewartsville Trail, a well-maintained gravel road that makes a straight shot up through an old cattle gate into the hills.

At exactly the halfway point of the ride, Stewartsville Trail intersects Contra Loma Trail on the right. Contra Loma Trail, just like Old Homestead Loop, Ridge Trail, and so on, is a great trail accessing the middle of the broad circuit described here. These trails can be strung together for additional loops/mileage or to cut the ride shorter by a few miles. If you do need to shorten your ride, you should probably avoid Ridge Trail, which you intersect at mile 5.2; it cuts a rugged path over the top of the ridgeline.

Once past Ridge Trail, Stewartsville Trail wraps around to the south of that predominant ridge and winds up in a wide plain that comes straight out of a Cormac McCarthy novel. The Old West sensation is interrupted only by the regular sound of small aircraft flying overhead, whose pilots are probably coming over from the Byron airport for a buzz of nearby Mount Diablo.

At the next three-way intersection, stay straight on Stewartsville Trail. Either of the two other options take you to an historic mine site. Make a left at the next intersection with Corcoran Mine Trail, shortly after which you cross a small puncheon over a streambed full of extremely happy trees and ride into the middle of a large stables area. Here the smooth gravel that has henceforth defined Stewartsville Trail ends in favor of the natural sandy soil. The next two left turns are Lower and Upper Oil Canyon Trails, respectively—make two rights to stay on Stewartsville Trail.

At mile 6.8 come to the Stewartsville backpack camp. There is an outhouse here, but you can't count on it being open. Otherwise this is a great shady spot to rest before tackling . . . the Wall.

The Wall has no trees. The Wall has no traction. The Wall has no respect for gravity. The Wall is under a mile long but feels like 10 miles. It's surprising there isn't more vegetation on the Wall for all of the sweat that must pour into that soil, or maybe it's just that most people avoid climbing this beast. Honestly though, you'd have just as hard a time climbing that steep bit of Lark Trail, and descending the Wall isn't the most fun, so the argument that this loop would be better in reverse is invalid. The views back down into the Stewartsville Townsite are pretty amazing—if you can see them through the sweat that will be streaming into your eyes, that is.

At the top, you find yourself back at the intersection with Carbondale Trail. Make the left and ride back down to the parking lot.

After the Ride

This area is awash with both taquerias and chain restaurants, and my money is definitely where the carnitas are. For the nearest taco stop, drive back down Somersville Road and make a left on Delta Fair Boulevard right before you pass under CA 4; in the Somersville Town Center you find Taqueria Salsa (phone (925) 778-9281). Another great option is Tres Salsa Taqueria (phone (925) 777-9777); hop back on CA 4 going east and exit on A Street, make a left onto A Street, and drive up to West 17th Street and find the restaurant on the left. If you're already heading back toward San Francisco, pop off on Railroad Avenue in Pittsburg, make a left, and drive four blocks (counting on your left) to find Morelia Taqueria (phone (925) 439-7070).

11

MORGAN TERRITORY REGIONAL PRESERVE: BIG SOUTHWEST LOOP

KEY AT-A-GLANCE INFORMATION

Length: 12.41 miles

Configuration: Figure-eight dog bone

Difficulty: 8/10; steep, prolonged climbs, but not too technical

Scenery: Views of Mount Diablo from the east

Exposure: Well-done

Ride traffic: Quiet on weekdays, low-to-medium on weekends

Riding time: 2–3 hours

Access: Free parking along Morgan Territory Road

Facilities: None; outhouse-style restroom early in the loop; no water

GPS TRAILHEAD COORDINATES (WGS 84)

UTM Zone 10S
Easting 0604840
Northing 4188080
Latitude N 37° 50' 9.7"
Longitude W 121° 48' 31.7"

In Brief

This longer of the two Morgan Territory rides described in this book is just shy of the longest possible loop available in the southwestern half of the park and actually dips into Mount Diablo State Park for a short stretch. That connectivity with another park means that the expansion possibilities are enormous. If you're looking for a more challenging ride, bring a lot of water and come prepared for long day of fast fire-road descents and hot, sun-drenched climbs in this stunning East Bay preserve.

Contact

Morgan Territory Regional Preserve
9401 Morgan Territory Road
Livermore, CA 94551
(925) 757-2620
www.ebparks.org/parks/morgan

Description

Standing at the coordinates on Morgan Territory Road and facing south, the trailhead will be on your right.

DIRECTIONS

From San Francisco, the southern route—55 miles (for the slightly shorter northern route, see the directions given in the next Morgan Territory ride). Head east across the Bay Bridge on Interstate 80. Once across the bridge, take the Interstate 580 East exit toward Downtown Oakland/Hayward-Stockton/CA 24. Drive 34.3 miles on I-580, then take the North Livermore Avenue exit toward downtown Livermore. Turn left so that you are heading north on North Livermore Avenue and drive just over 4 miles. North Livermore Avenue will turn left and become Manning Road. Shortly after, turn right onto Morgan Territory Road and drive 7.4 miles to the Highland Ridge trailheads—two green gates facing each other from the opposite sides of the road; park along either side.

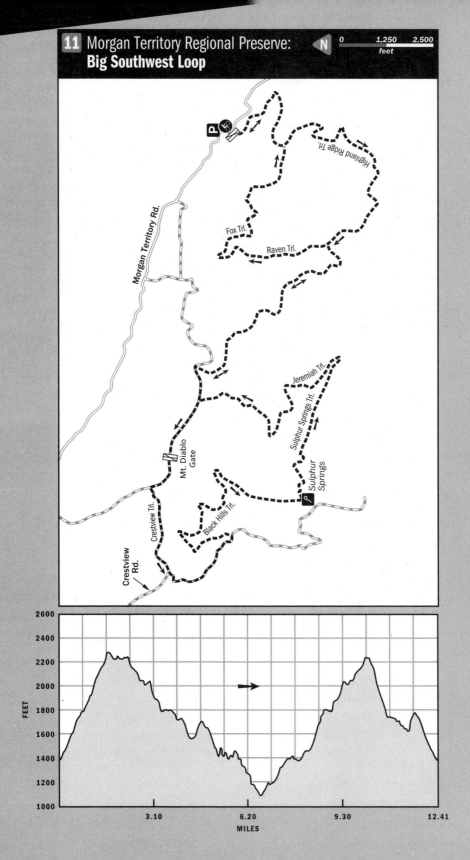

N

0   1,250   2,500
feet

Highland Ridge Trl.

Fox Trl.

Raven Trl.

Jeremiah Trl.

Sulphur Springs Trl.

Sulphur Springs

Mt. Diablo Gate

Crestview Trl.

Black Hills Trl.

Crestview Rd.

Morgan Territory Rd.

2600
2400
2200
2000
1800
1600
1400
1200
1000

FEET

3.10   6.20   9.30   12.41

MILES

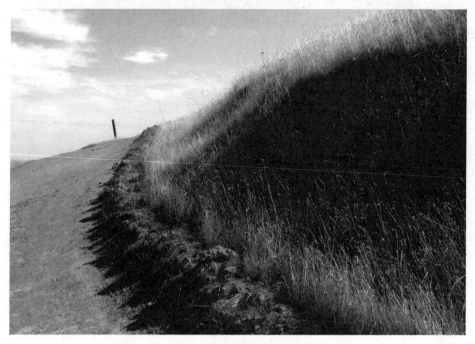

A post marks the top of this endless climb.

Highland Ridge Trail (aka the Bob Walker Regional Trail) cuts right across the road here and serves as the launch pad for both of the Morgan Territory rides in this book. Pass through the self-closing ranger gate and start climbing the fire road up the hill.

The initial climb up from the road gives a good indication of what to expect for the rest of the day: steep fire-road climbs. The day's average gradient is 10 percent, so if you came looking for Hatha Yoga and find this first climb a bit too Ashtanga, you might want to pop across Morgan Territory Road into the other side of the park and try the other ride (page 69), because the climbs on this one aren't going to get any easier. Pass through another self-closing gate, exit the trees, and 0.3 miles up the hill come to the first inter-section. Make a right, ride about 30 yards past a couple of withered old oaks, and make another right to keep on Highland Ridge Trail.

A third of a mile later, Raven Trail splits off right and dives down into the ravine; you'll climb back up this way later, but for now continue up the hill on Highland Ridge Trail. Just past this junction you'll find the only restrooms on the ride. From here the trail twists its way up the grassy hillside with the two peaks of Diablo looking on. After 1.6 miles straight up, the trail levels out on top of the ridge. The Bay Area's massive suburban growth hasn't quite reached this far east, and the long-ranging views you get from the ridgetops are gloriously unencumbered by human development.

As you crawl up on the ridge you can catch some of the stiff breezes rolling across from the west. The hills are predominantly bare, but there are strong clusters of live oaks, in addition to a few black oaks and buckeyes. The deciduous trees cut a truly stark profile against an early-morning winter sun, with long, skeletal shadows splaying out from their base, and the odd pair of ravens can really touch the scene with a pleasing Tim Burton kind of creepy.

Where the trail forks next, the left option is private territory and is usually locked behind a gate; continue right on Highland Ridge. The trail descends slightly for a half mile to the next junction with Raven Trail. Proceed left on Highland Ridge, passing through another gate (usually open), and go down the first real descent on this ride. It's a mile and a quarter of smooth fire road. Speeding along the top of the ridge, with clear sightlines and grass all around you, can begin to feel like one of the hawks that inhabit these skies searching out their small prey. The only thing this descent is missing is banked turns, so just go ahead and drift through the turns.

Make a left at the next, unmarked intersection to stay on Highland Ridge Trail and continue descending down the spine of the ridge. Just a breath past the last junction, Jeremiah Trail sneaks off behind the hillside on the left. You'll ride back up on this trail a bit later, but now continue straight on Highland Ridge Trail. A quarter mile down the ridge you'll come upon a closed gate with a big sign declaring that you are entering Mount Diablo State Park, which boosts the importance of this plain green park gate. In a way, though, transitioning from an East Bay regional park to Mount Diablo State Park does feel like transitioning between two different countries, as you'll find at the very next intersection.

As I've mention elsewhere in this book, the signage in Mount Diablo State Park borders on nonsensical and can be frustrating. The signs here do a great job of guiding you to dead ends and not a very good job of guiding you to recognizable landmarks in the park. At this intersection, despite what the sign may or may not say, make a left onto Crestview Trail. Crank it up and over the steep 45-yard climb and transition back into descent during which you'll pass unremarkably back into Morgan Territory. Unless you want to add a considerable amount of distance to this ride and push on to Mount Diablo, make two consecutive left turns on this descent.

Crestview Trail drops sharply off the ridge, makes a right, and then Ts into Black Hills Trail. You have a choice of going right or left on Black Hills Trail—both directions eventually take you to the same place, but your humble rider advocates the left option. Left cuts back across the hillside the way you've come but about 250 feet down the hillside, inside the tree line, which is fed by many separate small springs. Black Hills Trail is as mystical as its name indicates, dipping into a number of crevices formed by the seasonal springs. One of these in particular features a stunning, tiny little meadow framed by a huge, squat old live-oak tree. You'll often find a large buck hanging out in this area, occasionally sprawled out right on the trail itself.

The last bit of Black Hills Trail is a wild descent that follows the biggest of the small springs, crossing back and forth over the shallow bed like a snowboarder on a half-pipe (it is rather odd that the trail does this, in terms of environmental impact, but so it is). You'll often have to keep an eye out for large trail debris, branches, and such, since this trail is not regularly cleared. At mile 6.6, Black Hills Ts into Sulphur Springs Trail. Make a sharp left onto Sulphur Springs Trail and take a deep breath, because here's where the climbing resumes—1,100 some-odd feet of it, that is.

At the bottom of the Sulphur Springs climb, be sure to make a right at the intersection with Grizzly Trail, which is just impossibly steep to climb. Sulphur Springs Trail climbs under heavy tree cover, following yet another streambed up another crevice in the hills to a fairly unremarkable pond in the midst of a pretty remarkable little glen. The no-see-ums can be swarming on this climb here in early summer if there's any moisture left in the streams, but fortunately it's a fairly straight shot up a moderate grade, so if you've got any juice in the legs, just gun it and try to outrun them. Just below the pond, Jeremiah Trail forks off onto the other side of the streambed. The tiny little descent between trails is fun, but be careful because there are usually a few cows milling around in the shade.

Jeremiah Trail is a gorgeous slog, if there can be such a thing. This climb averages a 10 percent grade, twisting a bit as it climbs free of the trees and then, once out, cutting a direct path to the ridgetop along the grassy hillside. As gravity attacks your legs, immense views attack you from the west, and up ahead the trail disappears into a deep, blue sky. You have to look far off into the distance to catch a glimpse of any serious human development, so try not to look too hard.

At the top, make a right back onto Highland Ridge Trail and drag yourself back up the hill to the junction with Raven Trail, where you make a left. Raven Trail absolutely bombs straight down one of the finger ridges. If you get a chance—that is, if your brakes are still functioning—you can stop at points along this descent and take in the views, and maybe check out one heckuva big animal trap. This trap can only be designed for two things: grizzly bears or cougars, the thought of which sends chills down the spine.

Make the next right turn past the cage, onto Fox Trail, which cuts east across the face of the hill back toward Highland Ridge Trail. You'll pass over a somewhat disgusting stream full of bovine excrement, and then hit a steep climb. At the top of this climb, ignore the first left turn but take the second—at this point you should recognize the trail that you rode up on; it's just three-fourths of a mile back down to the car.

After the Ride

The best Mexican food nearby is in Livermore, and it is Casa Mexico at 4076 East Avenue. Drive back the way you came on Morgan Territory Road, and when you get back on North Livermore Avenue, pass under the freeway and drive 1.5 miles. Make a left onto East Avenue and drive a mile. The restaurant is on the north side of the street, so figure out how to turn around, or just park and walk over. They've got this orange margarita and excellent authentic Mexican food (phone (925) 371-0690).

12

KEY AT-A-GLANCE INFORMATION

Length: 6.55 miles

Configuration: 3-pronged loop

Difficulty: 3/10; a relaxed fire-road spin through the hills

Scenery: Ridgeline views of the Round Valley Regional Park

Exposure: Medium

Ride traffic: Quiet on weekdays, low-to-medium on weekends

Riding time: 0.75–1.75 hours

Access: Free parking along Morgan Territory Road

Facilities: Portable toilet midway through the ride; no water

MORGAN TERRITORY REGIONAL PRESERVE: VOLVON LOOP VARIATIONS

In Brief

Named for the small loop that forms the foundation for this ride, which in turn was named after one of the Native American tribes that used to inhabit the area, this ride makes good use of the side of the park that is to the northeast of Morgan Territory Road. The shorter of the two Morgan Territory rides featured in the book, this ride also has 2,000 feet less climbing. The topography in this half of the park is a little less severe than in the southwestern half, but the scenery and trail quality are equally superb. Many little additions and subtractions can be made to tailor this ride to your needs.

GPS TRAILHEAD COORDINATES (WGS 84)

UTM Zone 10S
Easting 0604774
Northing 4188042
Latitude N 37° 50' 8.1"
Longitude W 121° 48' 33.7"

DIRECTIONS

From San Francisco, the northern route—46 miles (for the slightly longer, southern route, see the directions given in the previous Morgan Territory ride). Head east across the Bay Bridge on Interstate 80. Once across the bridge, take the Interstate 580 East exit toward Downtown Oakland/Hayward-Stockton/CA 24 and immediately take the CA 24/Grover Shafter Freeway East exit toward Walnut Creek. Drive just over 13 miles to where CA 24 terminates at Interstate 680. Take the I-680 North exit toward Concord/Sacramento, keep right, and in just under a mile exit onto Ygnacio Valley Road. Drive 7.5 miles up Ygnacio Valley Road and turn right on Clayton Road. Drive 2.5 miles to Marsh Creek Road and turn right. Drive 3.4 miles down Marsh Creek and turn right onto Morgan Territory Road, which will take you 7.6 miles down a twisting, tree-shrouded one-lane road to the Highland Ridge trailheads—two green gates facing each other from opposite sides of the road; park along either side.

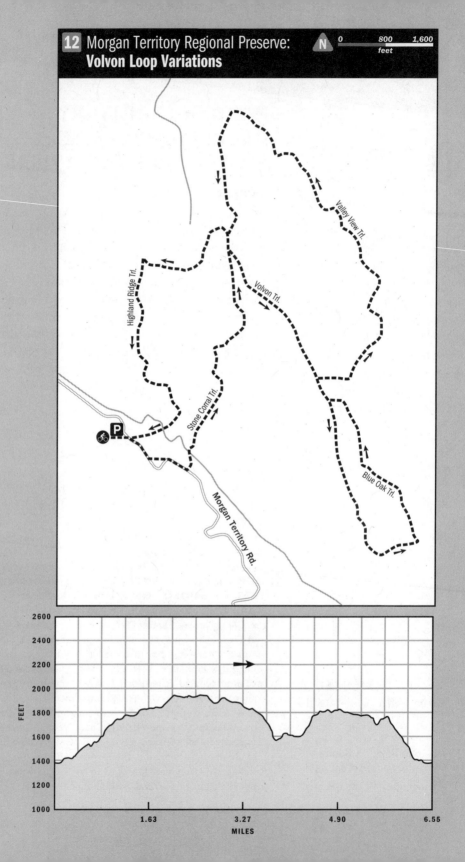

N

0   800   1,600
feet

Valley View Trl.

Highland Ridge Trl.

Volvon Trl.

Stone Corral Trl.

Blue Oak Trl.

P

Morgan Territory Rd.

2600
2400
2200
2000
1800
1600
1400
1200
1000

FEET

1.63   3.27   4.90   6.55
MILES

Contact

Morgan Territory Regional Preserve
9401 Morgan Territory Road
Livermore, CA 94551
(925) 757-2620
www.ebparks.org/parks/morgan

Description

The drive down Morgan Territory Road is adventure enough for one day, since much of it is a narrow, undivided one-lane road where other motorists and road cyclists are hiding around every shady blind turn. Presuming you followed the directions listed above and drove down from the north, the trailhead for this ride will be on your left as you arrive at the starting coordinates. The trailhead for the other Morgan Territory ride is right across the road, on the south side.

Saddle up and . . . well, first walk your bike through the narrow pedestrian walkway alongside the green gate, then saddle up and head out onto the Highland Ridge Trail, a fire road that descends slightly, going past a shady creek area—popular for picnics—and comes to the first junction, 220 yards from the car. Make a right here onto Stone Corral Trail, which is marked with the same type of signpost used throughout the East Bay parks system: a horizontal 4-by-4-inch square metal pipe with small, circular applications that feature arrows and trail names. These are difficult to read, particularly when they've become sun-faded, but with the rust-brown color of the metal, these signs do a good job of blending into the natural scenery.

Stone Corral Trail initiates the climbing, riding along the right-hand side of a small creek beneath a mix of bay, maple, and live-oak trees. The no-see-ums can be plentiful through here, unless the creek is dry toward the end of summer, and there is generally a large amount of scat on the trail from either coyotes or bobcats, all of which is a good indication that there is a healthy amount of vibrant wildlife in this remote part of the Bay Area.

The trail veers left and crosses the creek over a large culvert, then kicks up the climb a couple notches. Just where the tree cover breaks, a large oak frames the grassy hillside beyond, as if through Alice's looking glass. As you pass around this tree, you enter into what might possibly be the most beautiful meadow evah! This single view gives you a great idea of what urged a native Alabamian Jeremiah Morgan—the area's namesake—to settle here with his family and start a ranch back in the mid-1800s. You can see Coyote Trail cutting through the meadow to the trees on the far side; this is one of the few singletracks in the park, and it is off-limits to us.

Pass through a self-closing cattle gate and then over a small streambed that offers some exposed but tame rocks, and then through another gate and over a small tree-lined ridge, which lands you on an open grassy hillside below Bob Walker Ridge. Here you can see the current trail and your destination, Volvon Trail, laid out before you like ribbons over the undulating surface to where they meet at the top of a finger ridge. At this junction,

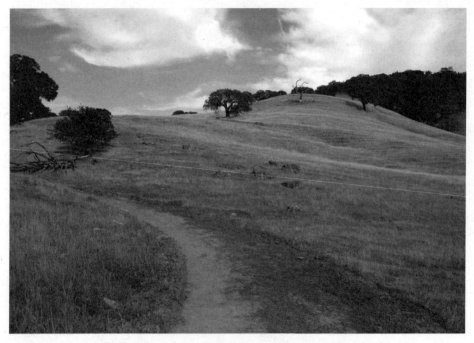

**Calmly rolling grassy hills exemplify the northern half
of the Morgan Territory Regional Preserve.**

make the sharp right turn onto Volvon Trail, but notice the other two trails that ricochet off the other side of this small ridge—you'll be back to enjoy these later on in the ride.

Volvon Trail cuts along the western face of Bob Walker Ridge, named for the photographer and environmentalist who favored Morgan Territory over all the other parks in the East Bay and in the 1990s worked as an activist to grow the park roughly 400 percent to its current size (5,000 acres). The ridge descends to meet the trail and at the next intersection, with Volvon Loop Trail, you find yourself on the ridgetop with good views back down the hillside from whence you came; trees prevent better views to the east. Make a right to stay on Volvon Trail.

Up next is Valley View Trail, where you'll find the ride's only restrooms (outhouse-style) on the other side of a cattle gate. Again, make a right to stay on Volvon Trail and continue to the south along the ridge. This is a fun, rolling section, where you can really turn on the juice and power along in a big gear through the oak trees, pretending that you're some barely controlled, rooster-tail-spitting, bright-orange Dodge Charger powered by Luke Duke. The trail makes a sweeping left turn (fish tail!!!) and comes to a three-way intersection; continue straight through the intersection and pick up Hummingbird Trail. However, if you're interested in expanding the ride, you could take the right onto Volvon Trail, which gradually climbs up to the Morgan Territory Road staging area, where you can find more restrooms and drinking water. A great addition to this ride is to take Volvon Trail, make a left onto Blue Oak Trail, a right onto Miwok, and a left onto Manzanita Trail, which would deposit you on Valley View Trail, adding upward of a mile to the overall distance.

Hummingbird Trail, at just 175 yards long, is as short as the bird is small, and it serves primarily as a connector trail. At the other end, make the sharp left onto Blue Oak Trail and ride back along the ridge. This stretch is just as hammer-fest fantastic as Volvon was in the other direction, and just a bit twistier. At the culmination of this small loop, make a right back onto Volvon and then another right onto Valley View, passing through the cattle gate (by the restrooms).

Grab a handful of brakes and head down the Valley View descent. Starting out at a respectable 12-percent grade through a medium oak forest, it finishes off with a downright gnarly 23 percent–grade drop through heavy trees down to a creek. That's 250 feet down in an eighth of a mile; paratroopers will do well on this descent. Sightlines are good, but traction can be slick with loose dirt and leaves, so watch out for other trail users—you don't want to spook a horse on this section. (Halfway down the descent you pass a trail on the right—this is Manzanita Trail from the expansion loop described earlier).

Valley View doesn't drop you all the way down into the valley but rather cuts along the hillside about 300 feet below the peak of the ridge. The trail gradually climbs up out of the tree line and then comes to fork. Down in the valley behind, you can catch a glimpse of the bright blue Los Vaqueros Reservoir. You can select either option at the fork—right is steeper, left is shallower. At the top, make a right onto Volvon Loop Trail. Volvon Loop Trail offers great views across the hills to Round Valley Regional Park as it wraps left around Bob Walker Ridge. Descend down to the intersection of Volvon and Stone Corral trails, which you'll remember from earlier. Make a right here onto Eagle Trail.

A third of a mile down the Eagle Trail descent, you come to an intersection with Hog Canyon Trail; make a left and climb up the steep climb to the intersection defined by the three trees that lean right, and then make another left onto Highland Ridge Trail. If unpredictable adventure is your thing, then both Hog Canyon and Eagle Trail are good options, as they careen off the East Bay parks map and into the unincorporated wilderness. If you've got enough juice in the tank you might just consider an exploration of one of these trails, otherwise Highland Ridge Trail is a ripping-fast descent straight down the face of the hill back to the car.

After the Ride

If you didn't pack a picnic to enjoy by the creek near the trailhead, your best bet for food is Casa Gourmet Burritos in the Walgreens parking lot in the town of Clayton, at 5435 Clayton Road. A few of the times I've been here on a Sunday, the restaurant has been closed, and they've always had a HELP WANTED sign in the window, but that situation may have changed. If you're planning on heading up on a Sunday, call ahead to find out if you'll be able to get your carne-asada fix or not (phone (925) 673-0908).

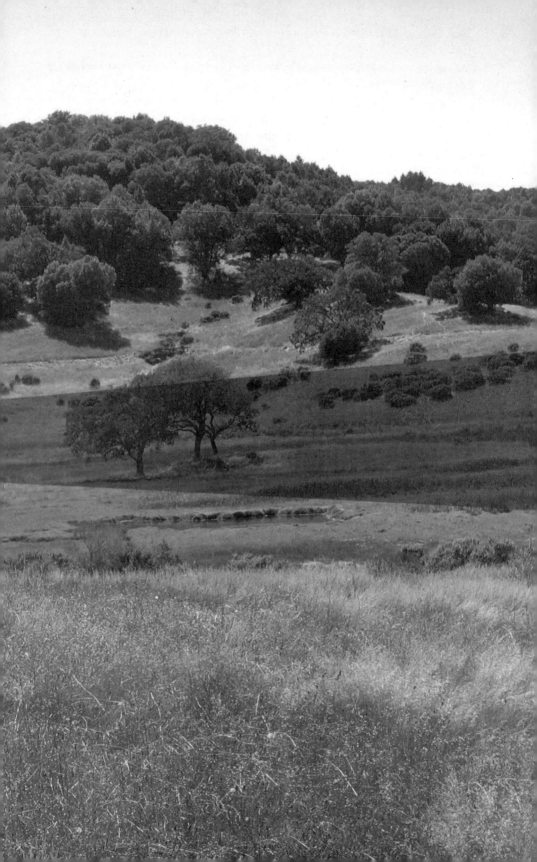

NORTH BAY

13

MARIN HEADLANDS: BIG SOUTHEAST LOOP WITH COASTAL TRAIL

KEY AT-A-GLANCE INFORMATION

Length: 10.84 miles

Configuration: Counterclockwise loop with 1.6-mile out-and-back

Difficulty: 7/10; moderately challenging terrain with a healthy amount of climbing

Scenery: Lush coastal scrub, grasslands, cypress groves, and great ridgeline views of the Bay Area

Exposure: High. There are a scant few shady spots on this loop, but coastal fogs generally keep the headlands very cool. Bring layers even in summer.

Ride traffic: Proximity to San Francisco ensures moderate traffic on evenings and weekends. Old Springs and Marincello trails consistently have most traffic.

Riding time: 2–2.75 hours

Access: Ample free parking along Conzelman Road, including in the small lot located at trailhead

Facilities: Midway through the ride, at the Tennessee Valley parking lot, there are restrooms and water fountains. It's best to bring your own water and food.

In Brief

The first of two loops in the Marin Headlands described in this book, this, the Southeastern loop, is popular with city mountain bikers as it is virtually right across the bridge and easy to ride to. The ride takes you over the ridge from Gerbode Valley to Tennessee Valley and back on a fun mix of singletracks, doubletracks, and fire roads. On a clear day, the ridgeline views, though incredible, are somewhat less impressive than those found in the northwestern region of the park, but the riding itself is more interesting. And, of course, this loop gives you the perfect excuse to ride/drive up Conzelman Road and check out its oft-photographed view of the bridge.

Contact

Marin Headlands
948 Fort Barry
Sausalito, CA 94965
(415) 331-1540
www.nps.gov/goga/marin-headlands.htm

GPS TRAILHEAD COORDINATES (WGS 84)

UTM Zone   10S
Easting   0544576
Northing   4187307
Latitude   N 37° 50' 2.20"
Longitude   W 122° 29' 36.43"

DIRECTIONS

By car: Drive north across the Golden Gate Bridge and exit at Alexander Avenue. Turn left at the fork onto Sausalito Lateral Road. Drive under the freeway and take the right turn up the hill just before you reenter the freeway. This is Conzelman Road.

By bike: Ride across the Golden Gate Bridge. If riding across the west side, you get spit out in parking lot right at the base of Conzelman Road. Ride out of the parking lot and turn left onto Conzelman Road. If riding across the east side, either use the footpath underneath the bridge or ride down Alexander Avenue and turn left under the freeway to get to Conzelman Road.

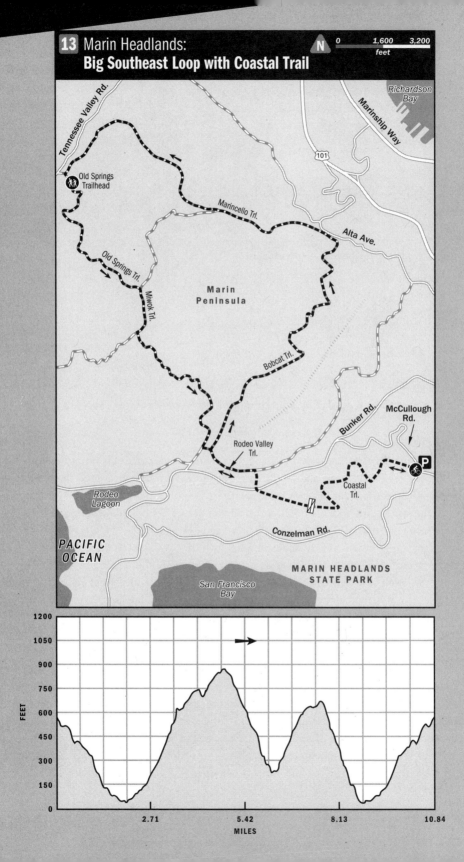

N

0   1,600   3,200
feet

Tennessee Valley Rd.

Richardson
Bay

Marinship Way

101

Old Springs
Trailhead

Marincello Trl.

Alta Ave.

Old Springs Trl.

Miwok Trl.

Marin
Peninsula

Bobcat Trl.

Bunker Rd.

McCullough
Rd.

P

Rodeo Valley
Trl.

Coastal
Trl.

Rodeo
Lagoon

Conzelman Rd.

PACIFIC
OCEAN

MARIN HEADLANDS
STATE PARK

San Francisco
Bay

1200
1050
900
750
600
450
300
150
0

FEET

2.71   5.42   8.13   10.84
MILES

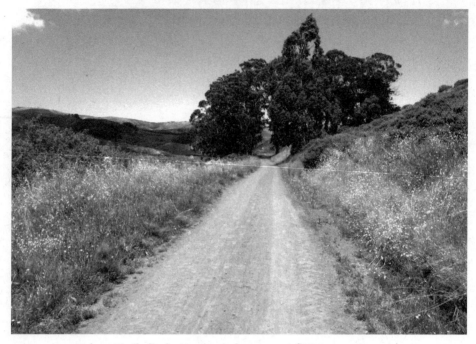

Bobcat Trail climbs up through a grove of Monterey cypress.

Description

Coastal Trail starts at the back of a small (less than six cars), gravel parking lot nestled in between Conzelman Road and McCullough Road. Make your way around the three-foot-wide gate, which is likely to be overgrown with bushes, and you're on the trail.

The ride begins with 1.2 miles of fun singletrack descending down through the same lush variety of coastal scrub that you had to squeeze through at the gate. In late spring and early summer, it can be like descending down through a leafy, green waterslide! It is really beautiful, but take care, as poison oak proliferates in this section of the headlands. The trail itself is a very nice, wide singletrack that is smooth except for some minor gulches running more or less down through the middle. In dry months these gulches range from just three to six inches deep and aren't very difficult to negotiate. Watch your speed on this downhill, though, as the turns are somewhat blind due to the exuberant flora. At the bottom of the descent, there is a larger gate that can creep up on you out of nowhere if you have a little too much speed going. Past the gate the trail widens into a fire road and runs for 0.1 mile through a small grassy valley before coming to paved Bunker Road.

To the left, Bunker Road runs out to the Marin Headlands Hostel, Rodeo Lagoon, and various beaches, while to the right, it heads inland toward Sausalito. Cross Bunker Road to the small dirt parking lot. Search in the bushes on the left-hand side of the lot for a small porthole that is the continuation of Coastal Trail. Drop into the trail and cross a puncheon. Then the trail turns right, and the bushes open up to grassland with a rustic wooden fence on the left.

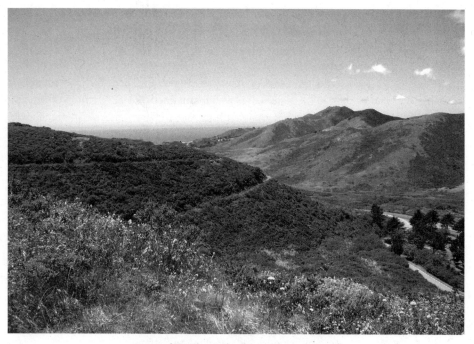

Coastal Trail overlooking Bunker Road

Just past the fence, turn left onto the intersecting Rodeo Valley Trail and ride this for 0.2 miles before turning right onto Bobcat Trail, which begins as a smooth, mild doubletrack climb up through the beautiful coastal grasslands. It passes through a stoic grove of Monterey cypress, after which it turns into a proper fire road.

After climbing steadily for 2.1 miles, you reach the top of the hill. Continue left on Bobcat Trail at the intersection. If it's a clear day, the views as you crest the hill open up. To your right, you can see down into Sausalito and across the bay, and to your left, you get a great view of the headlands and the ocean. From the ridge you drop down a fast 110-yard descent before the trail kicks back up.

About a mile past the last intersection, you will come to another intersection. Go right, continuing on Bobcat Trail (left is a nice detour to Hawk Lookout), and then the climb jets up and is made more difficult with both loose and fixed rocks. Choose a low gear and remain seated to maximize your traction through this section.

At the next intersection, split off right onto Marincello Trail. Here you will find more expansive views of the northern Bay Area, including notorious US 101 and its traffic that you, gladly, are *not* stuck in.

Marincello Trail begins descending at mile 5. This fun, twisty fire road descends with good visibility and ends at the bottom with a gate. Pass around the gate; to your right is the Tennessee Valley parking lot and to your left are Miwok Stables. If you're ambitious, you can connect here to the other headlands ride featured in the book (see page 81) for an amazing figure eight. If you're content with a single loop, go left toward the stables. You must get off the bike and walk through the stables, but it is only for a few hundred feet. Look for a small, two-horse stable off to the right, and Old Springs Trail will be just to the right of *that*. Don't dillydally too long in the stables area because the climb up Old Springs Trail is not forgiving of cold legs. Take a swig of energy drink and wait until the top of the hill to have a snack.

Old Springs Trail is an awesome doubletrack/singletrack. Because it is a popular multiuse trail, and so close to the stables, it is well maintained. Steeper sections of the trail have received rubber-mesh implants to help with impact and erosion. And let me tell you, some sections are steep! The trail winds sharply up the hill, ascending more than 300 feet in just 0.6 miles. Trail surface may be maintained, but the steepness and the odd camber of some of the turns keep this climb challenging. Kudos if you can climb the whole way without putting a foot down or simply passing out exhausted.

A small, wooden puncheon over a shallow gulch signals the top of the climb. If you're still breathing, take in some of the scenery from this vantage point, including a little piece of the beach visible from this angle. The trail flattens out along the top of the ridge, and there are a series of puncheons, which are designed to prevent user-aggravated erosion where the trail passes over small, seasonal waterways.

Take a right onto Miwok Trail, a fire road, which takes you a little farther along the ridge before it turns into a nice, fast descent. Be careful, as a couple of the turns have reduced visibility due to the way they cut around the hills, but otherwise enjoy yourself on this downhill. Near the bottom, when the trail begins to flatten out, keep a sharp eye for a trail to your left that is usually hidden by a combination of bushes, rider speed, and the angle at which it intersects Miwok Trail. Make a left onto this new trail, which is actually an old friend from the beginning of the ride: Bobcat Trail.

At the next intersection, make a right turn onto Rodeo Valley Trail again, and from here on you will be backtracking. Make the right turn back onto Coastal Trail after the wooden fence, cross through the dirt lot and Bunker Road, and then make the climb back up through the leafy, green waterslide to the trailhead.

After the Ride

Whether you're traveling by bike or by car, take Conzelman Road back down to the bottom of the hill, make a left onto Sausalito Lateral Road (right is the on-ramp for the Golden Gate Bridge), and follow this road under US 101 and down into Sausalito. You'll wind up on Bridgeway Road, which runs along the waterfront. It's very beautiful, and you could choose any of the expensive dining options along here, but I recommend following Bridgeway Road out of the shopping district to Spring Street, where you will find Saylor's South of the Border, Mexican cuisine and bar at 2009 Bridgeway Road (phone (415) 332-1512). They also have a fancier restaurant out on one of the piers, but lunches here start at $7.95, and happy hour features 99 cent tacos.

14

MARIN HEADLANDS: NORTHWEST LOOP FROM TENNESSEE VALLEY

KEY AT-A-GLANCE INFORMATION

Length: 5.31 miles

Configuration: Clockwise loop

Difficulty: 5/10; not technical and not long, but it does have a good climb to get the legs burning

Scenery: Amazing panoramic views of the northern Bay Area

Exposure: High. The last quarter of the ride is shaded, but the rest is wide open. Coastal fogs generally keep the headlands very cool, so bring layers, even in summer.

Ride traffic: The trail leading down to the beach bustles on a sunny day, but the rest of the park gets no more than the usual evening and weekend traffic.

Riding time: 1.25–2 hours

Access: Parking in the Tennessee Valley parking lot is free, and if the lot is full, there is plenty of parking along Tennessee Valley Road.

Facilities: Restrooms and water faucets at the parking lot

GPS TRAILHEAD COORDINATES (WGS 84)

UTM Zone 10S
Easting 0540622
Northing 4190015
Latitude N 37° 51' 40.30"
Longitude W 122° 32' 4.45"

In Brief

The shorter and more scenic northwest loop through the very scenic headlands, this book's second headlands ride takes you near Tennessee Beach, which functions as a sort of Stinson Beach overflow option for locals and clued-in (or time-strapped) tourists. The sight lines from the Green Gulch lookout point are unrivaled in the area . . . or are they? It's up to you to decide. The ride includes fire-road climbing with a snappy singletrack descent to finish the loop.

Contact

Marin Headlands
948 Fort Barry
Sausalito, CA 94965
(415) 331-1540
www.nps.gov/goga/marin-headlands.htm

DIRECTIONS

By car: From the Golden Gate Bridge, head north on US 101 and exit at CA 1 toward Mill Valley/Stinson Beach. In less than a mile, turn left onto Tennessee Valley Road. (Take care as traffic can be high, especially on weekends.) Drive up to the parking lot.

By bike: From the northeast corner of the Golden Gate Bridge, turn right onto Alexander Avenue and follow it down the hill to Bridgeway Road in Sausalito. Ride through Sausalito. You will pass A Bicycle Odyssey, which always has some incredible bike candy in stock, if you're interested. At US 101 on-ramp, look right for the separate paved bike lane on the other side of the fence (Mike's Bikes of Sausalito is also right here). Ride this for about a mile, under the freeway, and turn left before the wooden bridge. Ride until you come to the next wooden footbridge; Tennessee Valley Road is across CA 1 in this turn. Cross *carefully*. Ride up to the parking lot.

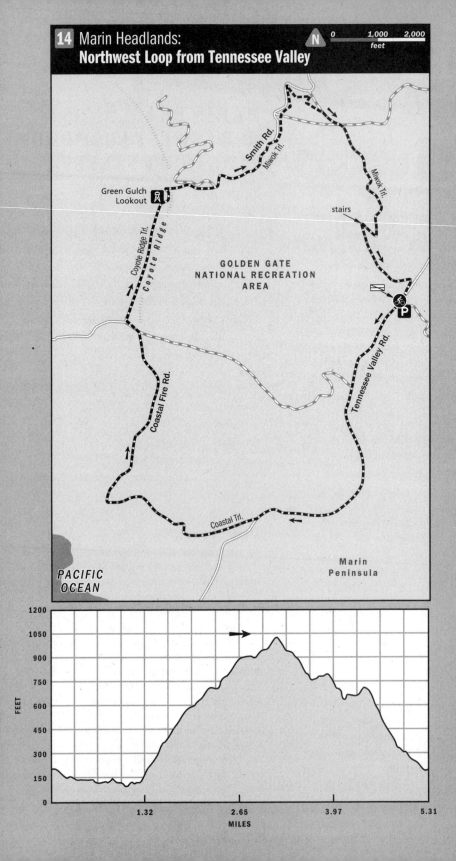

14 Marin Headlands:
Northwest Loop from Tennessee Valley

N

0   1,000   2,000
          feet

Smith Rd.

Miwok Trl.

Miwok Trl.

Green Gulch
Lookout

stairs

Coyote Ridge Trl.

Coyote Ridge

GOLDEN GATE
NATIONAL RECREATION
AREA

P

Coastal Fire Rd.

Tennessee Valley Rd.

Coastal Trl.

PACIFIC
OCEAN

Marin
Peninsula

1200
1050
900
750
600
450
300
150
0

FEET

1.32   2.65   3.97   5.31
                    MILES

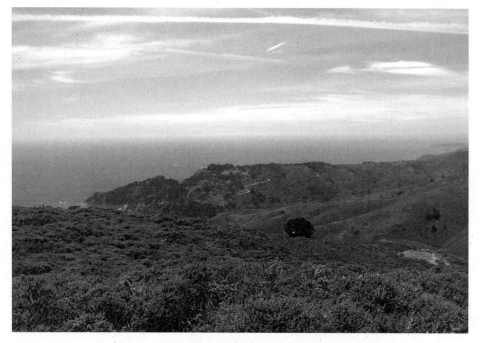

Looking out over the Pacific Ocean from Coyote Ridge

Description

Tennessee Valley Road continues through the gate at the end of the parking lot and down to the beach. Go around the gate and proceed down the road. There will be a lot of traffic on this section, as many people opt out of the hour-plus traffic leading to Stinson Beach and take the earlier cutoff that leads to Tennessee Beach. The extra traffic isn't a problem because the road here is so wide, and you'll be happy to note that 97 percent of this traffic disappears once you turn onto the trail proper. After 0.7 miles turn right onto a dirt fire road, descend another half mile, and make the right onto the well-marked Coastal Trail. Here's where the climbing begins.

Coastal Trail is a narrow fire road that winds up the coastal hillside, climbing 460 feet in 0.75 miles. The trail surface is well kept: not too loose, no favored lines. This is part of the California Coastal Trail project. At the time of writing, a little more than half of the proposed 1,200-mile trail running from Mexico up to Oregon is complete, but you will only ride this small portion of it today.

At the next intersection, Coastal Trail continues left but unfortunately becomes off-limits to bikes, so turn right onto the similarly named Coastal Fire Road and continue the beautiful climb up the hill. The hills are typical headlands fair: coastal scrub and grassland, practically no trees, and some beautiful rock outcroppings. As you climb higher, the hills gradually open up and let the surrounding views in.

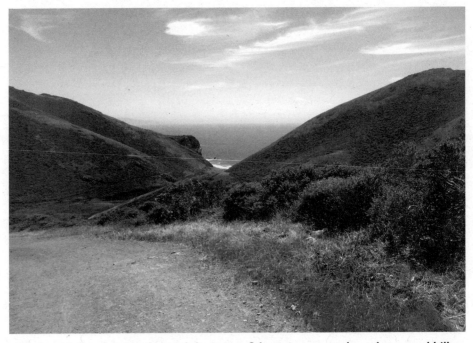

Tennessee Beach is just beyond the apex of these two coastal scrub-covered hills.

At the next intersection, continue left on Coastal Fire Road and after just a few hundred feet, make a right onto Coyote Ridge Trail. Stop here for a moment and take in the views of the ocean.

Coyote Ridge Trail offers more fire-road climbing along the ridge. The trail surface is a little looser, and there are usually one or two well-beaten paths that are easier to ride. Mile 2.1 signals the top of the hill. Look for a small, rocky trail jutting up sharply to the left. Make a small detour up there; you won't regret it.

This is just a lookout point, but it's a great place to have a snack. Green Gulch Trail actually begins here, but it's not accessible to bikes. From this vantage point, you have views all around. You can see down to Muir Beach, across to Sausalito, and the Golden Gate Bridge peeks at you through the hilltops. You will find absolutely incredible views on a clear day. Look on the ground and you'll see a one-foot diameter cement pad with a metal medallion sunk into it, which states that it is a Horizontal Control Mark from the National Geographic Survey. After your respite, head down and make a left back onto Coyote Ridge Trail, which rounds the corner and then descends steeply for a couple hundred feet. It's a straight descent, but a little loose, so keep your wits about you and your wheels under you.

Coyote Ridge Trail Ts into Miwok Trail at mile 2.34. Make a right onto Miwok and start descending. Miwok, at this point, is loose-pack fire road. Ignore any small singletracks peeling off Miwok because you will be descending this trail to the bottom. There are great views on the northwest side of the trail as you circle around that side of the mountain's peak, and once around the other side, you enter into the forest and the trail becomes steeper.

Watch your speed, as this section of trail is steep and usually loose. Make a right at the next intersection, staying on Miwok: left would take you down into a residential area. The trail remains pretty steep and loose through here, and the tree cover is dense, so visibility is slightly reduced in the shade. Keep your body weight back over the rear wheel and your attention on the front wheel.

When the trail flattens out and the trees open up, you come to a four-way intersection with County View Road cutting across Miwok Trail from left to right. Make a right, staying on Miwok Trail, which pops you over a little rise and back up on top of the ridge for more excellent views. Descending the ridge, the trail turns into a steep doubletrack made technical by small loose and fixed rocks. This is a very fun descent, and the trail gradually becomes skinnier and skinnier, eventually turning into a wide singletrack.

The most technical aspects of the entire ride come within a 1-mile section of this downhill. At mile 3.65 you will come to a very tight right-hand switchback that has the added difficulty of having an intricate system of wooden steps built into it. This section is very technical and should be approached very carefully. The steps are made out of six-inch square posts, so it would take a lot of suspension travel to completely smooth these out. The best line is around the outside of the steps. Just be careful as these steps could easily grab your front wheel and send you flying over the bars. Just after this there's another, tighter left-hand switchback, but this one is step-free. Then there is one more flight of steps, but this time they occur on a straight section of trail: the best line is to the left.

Reenter the forest for the downhill finale of the trail. This section is a fast, rolling singletrack, but be careful because you are likely to find more traffic at this point of the trail, since it is so close to the parking lot. Miwok Trail dumps you right back into the parking lot. If it's been a hot day, now would be a good time to head back down Tennessee Valley Trail and maybe check out the beach.

After the Ride

At the bottom of Tennessee Valley, make a left onto CA 1 and head just 100 yards up to the Dipsea Café located at 200 Shoreline Highway. They serve breakfast until 3 p.m.! What more could you want? Well, they also have a good lunch and dinner menu, and milkshakes (phone (415) 381-0298).

15

KEY AT-A-GLANCE INFORMATION

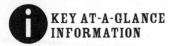

Length: 7.14 miles

Configuration: Clockwise loop

Difficulty: 5/10

Scenery: Thick redwoods and commanding views of the San Francisco Bay

Exposure: Medium

Ride traffic: High

Riding time: 1–1.75 hours

Access: Free parking

Facilities: Restrooms in parking lot, no water

GPS TRAILHEAD COORDINATES (WGS 84)

UTM Zone 10S
Easting 0537180
Northing 4195950
Latitude N 37° 54' 44.6"
Longitude W 122° 34' 38.1"

MOUNT TAMALPAIS STATE PARK: HOO-KOO-E-KOO AND OLD RAILROAD GRADE LOOP

In Brief

A condensed version of the other Mount Tamalpais ride described in this book, this loop is a very popular workout with area residents due to the ease of access from the Larkspur and Mill Valley neighborhoods. However, for out-of-town-visitor appeal I chose the Gravity Car fire road trailhead as the start point for this ride, but I also offer an explanation of how to access the far side of the loop.

Contact

Mount Tamalpais State Park
801 Panoramic Highway
Mill Valley, CA 94941
(415) 388-2070
www.parks.ca.gov/?page_id=471

Description

If you're interested in accessing this loop from the east side, then search out either Via Van Dyke Avenue or West Blithedale Avenue in Mill Valley, as both of these turn into fire roads and will land you on the loop. There are a few other obscure access points, such as Evergreen Drive

DIRECTIONS

By car: From San Francisco, head across the Golden Gate Bridge north on CA 101, drive 8.7 miles, and take the CA 1 exit toward Stinson Beach/Mill Valley. Drive 2.6 miles on CA 1 and take the slight right onto Panoramic Highway. Drive 2.6 miles up the hill and find the parking lot on the left, across from the Mountain Home Inn and Restaurant.

By bike: Much the same as the car directions above, although instead of riding CA 101 (illegal), head through the town of Sausalito and pick up the bike path at the north end of the town, ride that under the freeway overpass, and follow the path to the left to connect with CA 1. Take care on the stretch of CA 1, as it is a very tight and twisting two-lane road that is usually congested with traffic.

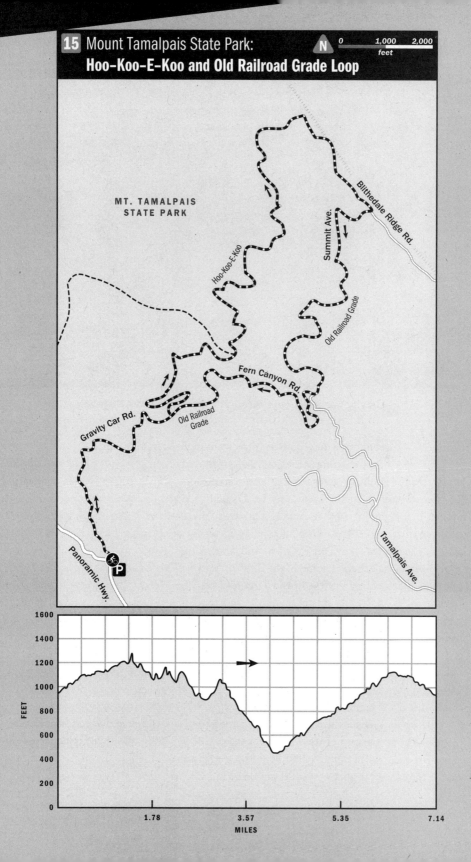

N

0   1,000   2,000
feet

MT. TAMALPAIS
STATE PARK

Blithedale Ridge Rd.

Summit Ave.

Hoo-Koo-E-Koo

Old Railroad Grade

Fern Canyon Rd.

Gravity Car Rd.

Old Railroad
Grade

Tamalpais Ave.

Panoramic Hwy.

FEET

1600
1400
1200
1000
800
600
400
200
0

1.78   3.57   5.35   7.14
MILES

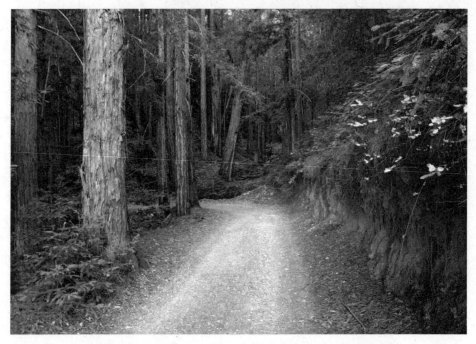

Gravity Car Road cuts through a ghostly redwood grove.

in Murray Park, but these don't connect directly to the loop in question.

For those of you starting at the prescribed trailhead on the west side, if the roadside lot off Panoramic Highway (across from the Mountain Home Inn) is full, you can drive into the Throckmorton Fire Station's driveway. At this point you should choose the middle of three options (left is the fire station, right is a private home; both are well marked), and this will land you in a small dirt parking lot right at the trailhead, 45 yards downhill from the fire station. This lot isn't listed on any maps and is rarely full.

From the gate at the far end of the little lot, strike out on Gravity Car fire road, a broad fire-protection road cut into the hillside. In the places where bits of the original hillside were left on the downhill right side of the trail, users have turned these innocuous bits of geography into little whoop-de-doos, by beating a trail along the tops of these small misshapen walls. There are no signs to detract one from enjoying these minor diversions, but experience indicates that park management probably frowns on them.

Gravity Car fire road climbs gradually through the trees for 0.8 miles and comes to a Y. Head left at the Y, and then make another left about 30 yards later, at which point you are on Old Railroad Grade fire road, heading north.

Old Railroad Grade fire road snakes up three switchbacks through the chaparral-covered hillside, and at the apex of the third switchback Hoo-Koo-E-Koo fire road splits off to the right. For such a wild name, Hoo-Koo-E-Koo is a relatively tame trail. From the junction it climbs for another eighth of a mile and then begins a very gradual (read flat) and smooth

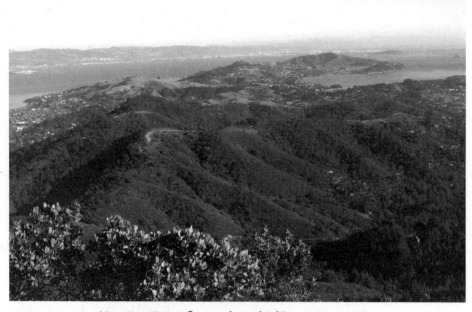

Hoo-Koo-E-Koo fire road overlooking Marin County

descent for the next 1.9 miles, dipping in and out of the contours of the hillside. Where the dense redwoods give way, you are greeted with great views across the bay to San Francisco.

As you churn along this gentle fire road, conversing with your ride mates or perhaps trying to roll the word *Hoo-Koo-E-Koo* into a catchy tune, you can admire some of the incredible singletracks that peel off here and there. Sadly, despite the fact that the sport was born here, mountain bikers have long ago worn out our welcome, and we are restricted to the basic fire-road fair while these fantastic singletracks taunt from all sides. They are great hiking trails, though, if you ever decide to leave the bike at home. Be warned that the regulations are very strict and bikes cannot even be pushed or carried along these trails; presence of a bike is enough for a ticket.

The next major intersection comes 3.1 miles into the ride, and it is where Hoo-Koo-E-Koo fire road meets Indian fire road and Blithedale Ridge fire road. There are good views from this spot, but if you want to crank up the views a notch, then turn left and ride 55 yards up to Indian fire road and check out the views from there. Had you come from Evergreen Drive in Murray Park, you would come down Indian fire road and picked up the loop here.

Turn right onto Blithedale Ridge fire road and head down the hill. The next mile is a very steep descent, with deep ruts and exposed bedrock thrown in to make things difficult. The turns also have loose, gravelly rocks that can easily cause wipeouts; be ready to drop your inside foot. This section of trail is the primary reason that the loop is rarely ridden in a counterclockwise direction, because trying to climb this beast is not all that enjoyable.

In the middle of the descent, half a mile past the last junction, make a right onto Old Railroad Grade, which drops off the ridge and dives for the trees. This is actually where Van Dyke Avenue would deposit you onto the loop had you come up from Mill Valley. The descent bottoms out in a mixed redwood-and-maple forest at 457 feet elevation, and this is where Old Railroad Grade meets West Blithedale Road (the other Mill Valley access point). Continue right on Old Railroad Grade, a well-maintained and even partially graveled fire road that begins a steady climb the other way across the mountain face.

Old Railroad Grade is very similar to Hoo-Koo-E-Koo fire road as it cuts across the face of the mountain in the other direction, but being a little lower on the hill, it experiences a little more of the encroachment of private homes, running right through the backyard of one in particular. Eventually the trail exits the trees and comes to an access gate, beyond which is the intersection of paved Summit Avenue and Fern Canyon Road (aka Old Railroad Grade). Turn right onto the latter street, which proceeds up the hill.

After suffering through a half mile of asphalt, Fern Road dead-ends at a couple of driveways. Old Railroad Grade continues, to the right, passing through the nearest home's backyard. Three-fourths of a mile later brings you back to Gravity Car fire road; make a left to get back to the parking lot.

After the Ride

Within walking distance of the Gravity Car trailhead, at 810 Panoramic Highway, is the Mountain Home Inn. The restaurant's menu is limited, but the food is excellent. Even if not hungry, many people come here just to enjoy a beer or glass of wine on the back deck, which has a view that you might normally ride hours for. You might even consider an overnight stay in one of the rooms, which would give you an extra day on Mount Tamalpais, time enough to tackle Eldridge Grade (phone (415) 381-9000).

16

KEY AT-A-GLANCE INFORMATION

Length: 15.19 miles

Configuration: Clockwise loop

Difficulty: 10/10. There is a lot of climbing, but it's the rocks that boost this to 10.

Scenery: Chaparal, redwoods, lakes, and 2,500-foot views

Exposure: Medium-well

Ride traffic: High; it is, after all, Mount Tamalpais

Riding time: 2–3.5 hours

Access: Free parking in Rock Spring parking lot on East Ridgecrest Boulevard

Facilities: Restrooms, no drinking water. Carry a lot of water on this ride.

GPS TRAILHEAD COORDINATES (WGS 84)

UTM Zone 10S
Easting 0534170
Northing 4195780
Latitude N 37° 54' 38.9"
Longitude W 122° 36' 39.1"

MOUNT TAMALPAIS STATE PARK: NORTHERN LOOP— ROCK SPRING ROAD TO ELDRIDGE GRADE VIA BON TEMPE LAKE

In Brief

Starting from East Ridgecrest Boulevard, this ride follows a rocky descent down the Lagunitas Rock Springs fire road to Alpine and Bon Tempe lakes, circling back on the far side of the lakes to the legendary Eldridge Grade fire road. Just as Lombard Street must be driven, the De Young visited, and Golden Gate Park frolicked in, so too must Mount Tamalpais be ridden, at least once. For experienced, fit riders living in or visiting the Bay Area, this ride offers a satiating amount of climbing, technical challenges, and visual stimulation.

Contact

Mount Tamalpais State Park
801 Panoramic Highway
Mill Valley, CA 94941
(415) 388-2070; www.parks.ca.gov/?page_id=471

DIRECTIONS

By car: From San Francisco, head across the Golden Gate Bridge north on CA 101, drive 8.7 miles, and take the CA 1 exit toward Stinson Beach/Mill Valley. Drive 2.6 miles on CA 1 and take the slight right onto Panoramic Highway, drive 5.3 miles up the hill, and make a right onto Pan Toll Road. Where Pan Toll Road Ts into East Ridgecrest Boulevard, find the parking lot. You can also turn right onto East Ridgecrest Boulevard and drive another 0.2 miles to a smaller dirt lot directly across from the trailhead.

By bike: Much the same as the car directions above, although instead of riding CA 101 (illegal), head through the town of Sausalito and pick up the bike path at the north end of the town, ride that under the freeway overpass, and follow the path to the left to connect with CA 1. Take care on the stretch of CA 1, as it is a very tight and twisting two-lane road that is usually congested with traffic.

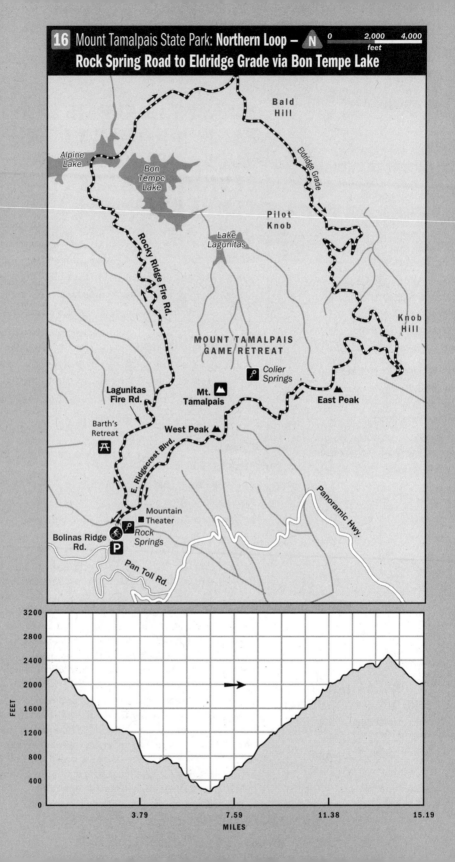

Description

If you parked in the Rock Spring parking lot at the top of Pan Toll Road, then grab your bike and ride uphill on East Ridgecrest Boulevard for 0.4 miles and look for a fire road and brown park gate on your left. Beyond the gate, in the sunny field on the right side of the road, see an old hand-carved wooden sign declaring that this is the Lagunitas Rock Springs fire road (otherwise known as Rock Springs Lagunitas fire road in park literature, and referred to as the Lagunitas fire road for the remainder of the piece—both for brevity's sake and because nearby Lagunitas Brewery makes some mighty fine beers).

Lagunitas fire road starts out smooth, climbing for the first 35 yards before cresting the ridge and beginning a long stair-stepping descent down to the lakes. A good rule of thumb for riding in Mount Tamalpais is to avoid all singletracks. A 1996 court ruling (read here: http://classweb. gmu.edu/jkozlows/marin.htm)

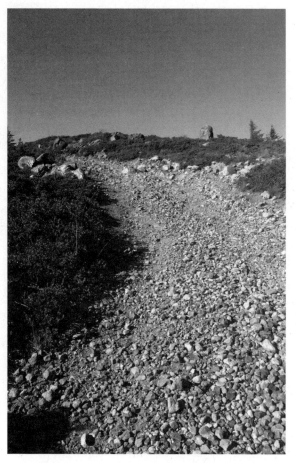

The pulverizing Rocky Ridge fire road rock garden

drastically cut down mountain bike access in the park, and the climate remains tumultuous. There are one or two singletracks still open to mountain bikes, but this ride doesn't touch any of them. Since there are no singletracks included in this jaunt, all directions preclude the existence of these trails (for example, a five-way intersection that includes two singletracks will be referred to as a three-way intersection). Be warned that the regulations are very strict and bikes cannot even be pushed or carried along trails that are deemed no bikes—presence of a bike is enough for an expensive ticket.

Over the ridge, descending through a pine forest, the fire road becomes slightly coarser with loose rocks and roots. Just under a mile into the ride, you come to a junction with Laurel Dell fire road: make a right to continue on Lagunitas fire road, which flattens out and skirts around the right edge of Potrero Meadow. Then you reenter the woods, and the fire road gets friskier, with some good twists to avoid the pines and bay trees as well as some man-made

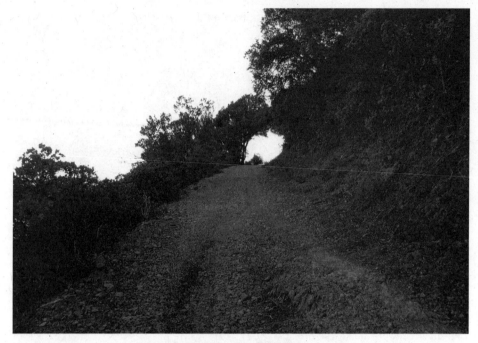

A portal near the top of Eldridge Grade

water control dips, off of which you can grab a little 15 mph air. Make a right at the intersection with Lagoon fire road, continuing on Lagunitas fire road, which trades woods for chaparral. After a brief climb, the trail enters a small wood. Make a 170-degree left turn onto Rocky Ridge fire road as Lagunitas fire road continues straight down the hill.

From a technical standpoint, Rocky Ridge fire road is the highlight of the first half of the ride. This is an awesomely steep and rugged descent with large rocks and deep ruts to keep you alert, fingers primed on the brake levers, and eyes scanning for the best line through the rough stuff. It's a color-changing trail, too, going from brown to red to granite gray over the course of its almost 2-mile length. At the bottom of the descent, a swooping right-hander leads into the *coup de grâce:* a 55-yard climb up through a massive rock garden. Click it into a medium gear and slog through the loose, little rocks at the bottom of the climb, then try to get a downshift in at the transition to the larger, fixed-rock upper section. Once over top, pass through a stand of trees and drop down onto the dam that separates Bon Tempe and Alpine lakes.

Ride across the dam and turn left into the Alpine Road parking lot where you find a portable toilet. There are no drinking fountains, which is ironic since these are the lands belonging to the Marin Municipal Water District. It's this sort of magnanimity that's prevented the BART system from making its much needed way up to the North Bay.

From the Alpine Lake parking lot, make a right onto the gravel Alpine Road, ride up to Sky Oaks Road, which is paved, and make a right. Just 22 yards up Sky Oaks Road, look for a wood gate leading to a fire road on the left. This is Elliot Trail, but the signpost indicates

Shaver Grade and Five Corners, with arrows. Ride down this fire road and come to Five Corners, a busy intersection of trails and a popular spot to take a break and enjoy some sun. Find the trail marked Shaver Grade where it exits out the other side of this circle of trailheads and continue the mellow descent through a forest of dramatic bay and maple trees and stolid, straight pines, making a left at the next fork with Concrete Pipe Road.

Next up you come to a four-way intersection at a low elevation of 209 feet. Just to keep things in perspective, you started at an elevation of 2,200 feet 6.6 miles ago, and you will be climbing up to 2,500 feet elevation in the next 5+ miles up Eldridge Grade. Shaver Grade continues straight down the hill while Fish Grade fire road is a hard right, shooting straight back up the hill toward the lakes (not a fun one to climb). Take the soft right onto Lower Eldridge Grade and begin crankin' them pedals. Actually there's no hurry, especially in late fall, when the maple leaves paint the area in yellows and oranges; it's a visual feast. Speaking of food, if you haven't eaten in awhile, you should eat at the base of this climb, otherwise you will definitely bonk on the way up.

It's easy to follow Eldridge Grade up the hill; all of the intersections are well marked, and as long as you follow the signs and keep ascending, you're doing all right. The trail is fairly smooth for the most part, switchbacking its way up the eastern face of Mount Tamalpais at a consistent 9 to 10 percent gradient, with the peak looming overhead. The scene from the Wheeler Trail switchback (third from the top) actually rivals the beauty of the famed switchback on Harkins Ridge Trail in the Purisima Creek Redwoods Open Space Park; it really depends on whether you prefer a city or a forest backdrop. There's something about a roadway doubled back on itself high on a hillside above a scenic valley floor that's exquisite in my mind.

Eldridge Grade makes a broad loop around the peak to the north, and the last mile of trail is very rough and rocky, with spots nearly as difficult as Rocky Ridge fire road. You and your shattered legs get spat out onto East Ridgecrest Boulevard. Turning right will take you back down to the car in just over one—paved—mile. However, it's obligatory to turn left and climb the final 0.25 miles up to the East Peak parking lot and visitor center on top of the mountain. If your bottles have been dry since the bottom of the mountain, the water fountain here might just be the greatest attraction for you. Assuming you're not deliriously dehydrated, and it's a clear day, though, you might just want to check out the view.

After the Ride

Hop in the car and drive back down Pan Toll Road, but instead of turning left on Panoramic Highway to head back toward San Francisco, turn right and drive down to the little town of Stinson Beach to check out the Sand Dollar Restaurant, right in the middle of town at 3458 CA 1. More Jerry Garcia than Celine Dion, this is a great place for burgers and brewskies, and especially on the nights when they feature live music (phone (415) 868-0434).

17

CHINA CAMP STATE PARK: SHORELINE TRAIL AND OAK RIDGE LOOP

KEY AT-A-GLANCE INFORMATION

Length: 6.01 miles

Configuration: Clockwise balloon

Difficulty: 7/10; moderately technical with a long, gradual climb and steep downhill

Scenery: Potpourri of classic Bay Area views

Exposure: Medium

Ride traffic: High—a great park in a high-population area translates to high traffic.

Riding time: 2–3 hours

Access: Free parking in neighborhood off Biscayne Drive

Facilities: None at trailhead or on the trail itself, but you can take short detours from the loop to find facilities at Bullhead Flat and China Camp Village.

In Brief

This ride is a loop comprised almost entirely of fantastic, switchbacky singletrack that pops in and out of incredible oak-dominated forest. Rather than fight the weekend parking-lot havoc that can be China Camp, I suggest a somewhat nontraditional starting point in the neighborhood off Biscayne Drive.

Contact

North San Pedro Road
San Rafael, CA 94901
(415) 456-0766
www.parks.ca.gov/?page_id=466

Description

Point San Pedro Road makes a big horseshoe loop east off US 101, encompassing China Camp State Park in its circuit. Biscayne Drive quietly peels off Point San Pedro Road at the farthest point from US 101, slipping into the neighborhood that is tucked away in the southeast corner of the park. Shoreline Trailhead is about 30 yards past the intersection on the right-hand side of the road and just 45 feet above sea level. It's easily identifiable due to the gate and obvious trail cutting through and up the grassy hill. Be sure not to park at the red curbs that extend a couple hundred feet on either side of the trailhead.

Shoreline Trail begins as a doubletrack that shoots up a short, little grassy hill toward a eucalyptus stand.

GPS TRAILHEAD COORDINATES (WGS 84)

UTM Zone 10S
Easting 0547669
Northing 4205293
Latitude N 37° 59' 45.18"
Longitude W 122° 27' 25.53"

DIRECTIONS

From the Golden Gate Bridge, head approximately 11.5 miles north on US 101 to the Central San Rafael exit. Turn right off the exit onto Second Street, drive an eighth of a mile, and merge onto Third Street, heading east. Third Street turns into Point San Pedro Road, and in 4 miles, make a left onto Biscayne Drive.

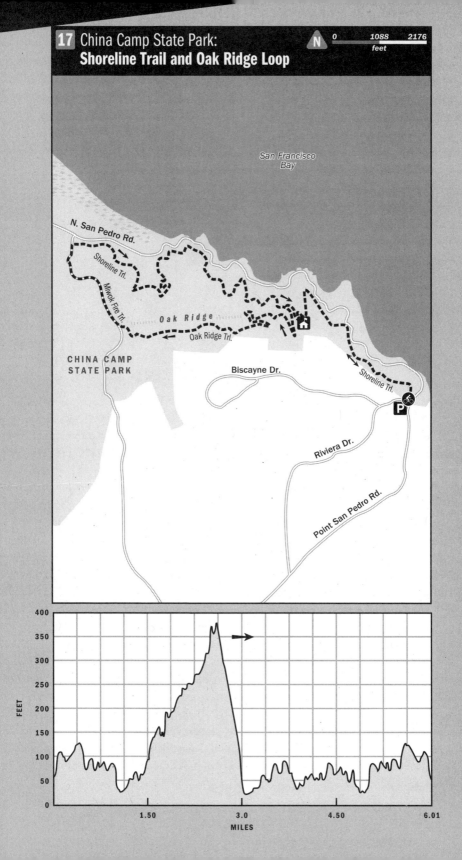

San Francisco
Bay

N. San Pedro Rd.

Shoreline Trl.

Miwok Fire Trl.

Oak Ridge

Oak Ridge Trl.

CHINA CAMP
STATE PARK

Biscayne Dr.

Shoreline Trl.

P

Riviera Dr.

Point San Pedro Rd.

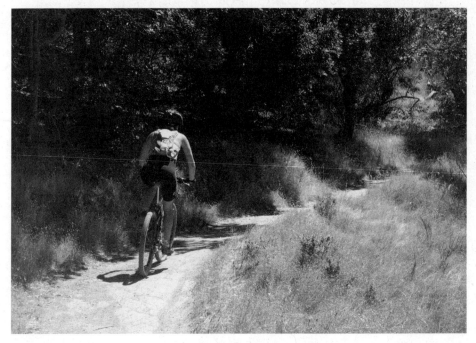

Powering along Shoreline Trail

There is coyote brush on either side of this little climb, and it's not uncommon to see coyote scat on this part of the trail. You might even scare up a deer or two, braving the coyotes to cool in the shade of the bushes during the day.

At the top of the little hill, from beneath the shade of the eucalyptus trees, you can see majestic Mount Tamalpais towering above all else to the southwest. As you continue along the low ridge beyond the trees, the views of the bay open up. They're beautiful, but there's no need to stop and enjoy these particular views, since Shoreline Trail affords plenty of them.

The trail turns into singletrack, and after an eighth of a mile, you come to an intersection; take the left option, as right takes you to the China Camp Village parking lot. Here, at the base of a medium-size live oak, is a trail sign indicating the very strict speed limits in the park: 5 mph around turns or when passing, and 15 mph top speed at all times. And it's no joke—the park can be very busy, and rangers patrol regularly.

Just past the sign is an unmarked three-way fork. Go right on Shoreline Trail. This is where the hill starts to rise and Shoreline slips around on the right side. The trail heads toward a large stand of bay trees, past a treeless hillside covered with ferns that are largely baked yellow and orange in the summer sun intermixed with poison oak, coyote brush, and some berry vines.

Once in the trees, the bug population explodes, and for some reason it's particularly high where the trail goes over a little bridge. Don't linger here, unless you're fond of horsefly and mosquito bites or wasp stings. Just try not to break the 15 mph speed limit as you flee the area.

The next fork features a bench overlooking the bay, should you care to rest already. Make a right at the fork, continuing on Shoreline Trail, which enters into a small forest of madronas and live oaks. There's poison oak hanging from the branches and, in summer and fall, the bright red leaves dot the ground. The trail winds and dips in and out of these shady tree clusters. There are some surprisingly large trees in this park, including one that arches over the trail like the gate to John Muir's outdoor palace.

Shoreline Trail curves around the ridge at Five Pines Point, changing direction from northwest to southwest. The shore of the bay becomes marshy past Five Pines Point, and breeding in amongst the scenic reeds are hundreds of thousands of mosquitoes. Yes, they do find their way the few dozen yards up to the trail. It's not such a problem at riding speed, but if you stop, you will be bombarded.

The trail descends and comes to a paved road and ranger station, another place to stop for restroom or water facilities. Cross the road directly to where Shoreline Trail continues to the other side. The trail, which cuts to the right up the hillside, is reinforced to prevent washing out. Immediately you come to a left-hand switchback. There are wooden railings running along the trail at this point to discourage trail shortcutting.

Zipping up through the shady woods, Shoreline Trail goes through a couple more switchbacks, the third of which doubles as a trail junction. This is where Shoreline Trail meets Oak Ridge Trail, with the former bursting out the end of the switchback and continuing off to the right, while Oak Ridge Trail completes the switchback, coming down off the hill from the left. Go left onto Oak Ridge Trail and continue the progression up the hill. Make note of this intersection, because you will be returning to it on Shoreline Trail later.

Oak Ridge Trail is a singletrack that twists its way up the forested hillside. Sunk in the trees, you lose sight of the bay, but there is plenty of visual excitement with oak, bay, and madrona trees cascading around at all angles. It feels a lot like being inside a jungle gym, with sections of trail visible below and above through the twisty limbs.

Just before your odometer clicks over 2 miles, Oak Ridge Trail crosses the McNears fire trail for the first of two times within a half mile. Proceed straight through on Oak Ridge Trail. Through here the trees relent a bit, and you find great views to the south all the way to the San Francisco skyline. You can also see Treasure Island and the Bay Bridge in the background, with the Richmond Bridge in the foreground.

The singletrack continues to wind along the southern hillside, and then you come to the second intersection with the McNears fire trail, which takes the exposed route along the ridgetop to the left, while you go right, disappearing back into the woods. There are trail markers at the intersections.

This is the last bit of serious climbing for the ride, and it's all shaded. In late summer, one of the plants that preponderates along the side of the trail goes to seed and the seeds float on wispy cottonlike pods, which often wind up coating the trail like some sort of freak subcanopy snowstorm.

Oak Ridge Trail spits you out of the trees and onto the Miwok fire trail at mile 2.6. This is also the highest elevation point on the ride at 380 feet. Turn right onto Miwok fire trail and prepare yourself for a very steep descent straight down off the ridge. This is the triple black diamond of the park, and other than the slight cant to the left and some turns near the bottom, it follows a very direct route to the bottom of the hill.

Oak Ridge Trail is very wide and not especially rough, aside from a rut running down the right-hand (in the downhill direction) side of the trail. The steepness of the trail will test your ability to stay under the speed limit, but fortunately visibility is high enough to mitigate any issues that might arise with other trail users. At the bottom there is a wooden gate that is usually closed with a pedestrian access at the side, and once on the other side, you find yourself at Miwok Meadows.

Twenty-two yards past the gate is a trail junction, and here you can catch a glimpse of the meadow, which is a marshy area featuring an amalgamation of various greens and yellows sunk into the grassy hillsides. There is the tiniest grassy knoll peaking up out of the center of the marshy meadow where three live oaks live. If you want to experience the meadow up close, you can go left, which will take you to the Miwok Meadows day-use area. For this ride, though, head right onto Shoreline Trail.

This is the other 1.6-mile section of Shoreline Trail that takes you back to the junction with Oak Ridge Trail. It's more of the same excellent, rolling and twisting singletrack featured throughout the ride. Initially exposed with great views of the bay and the marsh on the left, the trail then pops into the trees, and at mile 3.7 makes use of short wooden bridges to cross a couple of small creeks. In addition to the bridges, there are some really technical switchbacks within this section.

At mile 3.9 the trail jogs right to avoid a gigantic live-oak tree, which would be a great shady rest spot except that there is nowhere to sit. At mile 4.75, you come to the fork where you took Oak Ridge Trail to the top of the hill earlier. To make it back to the car, just go left at the fork and retrace your tracks along Shoreline Trail, 1.25 miles back to the car.

After the Ride

Head back to US 101 and find Taqueria San Jose, tucked underneath the freeway, away from some of the pretentiousness of San Rafael, at 615 Fourth Street. This is a very traditional taqueria where you can get uber-cheesy nachos, soft tacos, tacos dorados, or "wet" burritos—smothered in enchilada sauce—and wash them down with imported beers (phone (415) 455-0999).

18

BOLINAS RIDGE TRAIL: BOLINAS RIDGE OUT-AND-BACK

KEY AT-A-GLANCE INFORMATION

Length: 22.8 miles, 11.4 miles one-way

Configuration: Out-and-back

Difficulty: 7/10. Although not very technical, this ride *is* very long.

Scenery: A survey of Northern California microclimates; great bird's-eye view of Stinson Beach

Exposure: Medium-rare; tree cover for a wee more than half of the ride

Ride traffic: Light. You will see more traffic at either end of this long stretch of trail, while only the most avid enthusiast should attempt the middle.

Riding time: 3.5–5 hours

Access: Limited free roadside parking at either end of the trail

Facilities: None

In Brief

Bolinas Ridge Trail is a long, point-to-point affair that spans the just more than 11-mile gap between Fairfax-Bolinas Road to the south and Sir Francis Drake Boulevard to the north. The ride described here is an out-and-back affair beginning at and returning to Sir Francis Drake Boulevard. However, if you're not up for a 23-mile mountain bike ride, you can do the trail in two halves, or perhaps have someone pick you up at one end, for a true point-to-point experience.

Description

Starting at the gate on Sir Francis Drake Boulevard, you enter through a tight, serpentine pedestrian walkway designed to keep the cows in. The gate is relatively low, so most will have no problem hoisting their bikes over. Ride past the Bolinas Ridge Trailhead sign and go about

DIRECTIONS

There is an inland and a coastal route to reach the start of this ride. For the coastal route, head north on US 101 from the Golden Gate Bridge and take the CA 1/Stinson Beach exit. Head over the hill to Stinson Beach and from there, head up CA 1 14 miles to Olema. In Olema make a right onto Sir Francis Drake Boulevard and drive 1 mile to the trailhead. Because it is popular with tourists and a much less direct route, the coastal route will take longer than the inland route.

For the inland route, take US 101 north from the Golden Gate Bridge 11.5 miles north to San Rafael. Take the Central San Rafael exit and make a left onto Fourth Street. Drive west on Fourth Street until it turns into Red Hill Avenue, and then make a right onto Sir Francis Drake Boulevard. From the intersection of Red Hill Avenue and Sir Francis Drake Boulevard, drive 16 miles to the trailhead. Both routes make for a beautiful drive.

GPS TRAILHEAD COORDINATES (WGS 84)

UTM Zone 10S
Easting 0530090
Northing 4210750
Latitude N 37° 56' 22.6"
Longitude W 122° 39' 26.9"

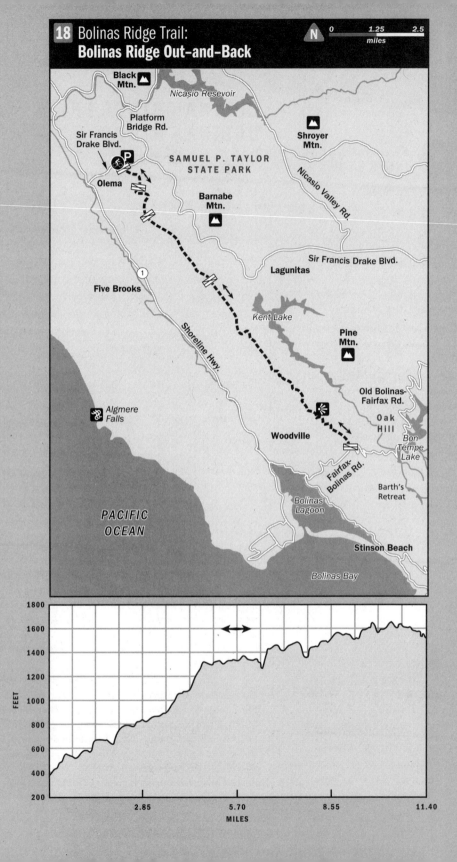

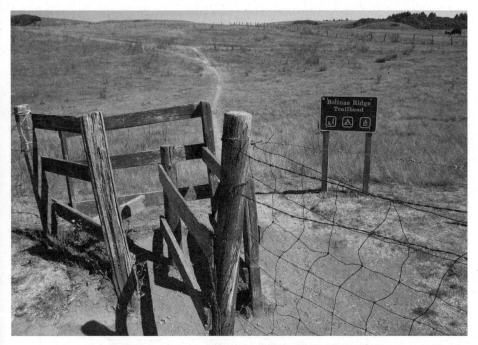

To embark, hoist your bike over the barbed-wire fence . . .

25 yards up a singletrack through an open grassy field to the actual trail, which is a fire road.

Right away the fire road starts with a mild climb, up through the open grassland toward a dense cluster of live oaks hugging the north face of a small hill. From a distance, this cluster of trees looks oddly cultivated, like a carved hedgerow in front of a fancy estate home. As you approach, though, this small wood takes perspective, and you begin to notice the rings of cattle trails surrounding the woods. On a hot day, you'll actually find that a number of cattle have taken shelter in these trees to get away from the sun, as though it were some lumpy green barn.

Continuing its ascent through some large rock formations standing like sentries in the hills, the trail levels out where it passes by more trees. At mile 1.1 you come to another cattle gate with one of those snaky human passageways. From here you can look north and catch a glimpse of the southern tip of Tomales Bay off in the distance.

Another mile brings another gate, but this one is metal and features a simple chain-latch system that users must open and close behind them, on the honor system. Beyond this gate the grass has been winning the battle against trail traffic, overgrowing the fire road, whittling it down so that it looks like a singletrack.

Hit another one of the wooden serpentine gates at mile 3, beyond which the trail climbs up a grassy hill for another 0.6 miles past a man-made watering hole for the cattle and then up onto the ridge. The last bit of this climb is steep, rocky, and rutted. There are singletracks snaking off in all directions through here; these aren't legal trails, but rather trails made by the cattle coming in from all around to slake their thirst at the small man-made pond.

The ridge above the pond is one of the more scenic parts of the ride. Initially you are greeted with a semi-truck-sized rock outcropping with a small and withered old tree growing out of the top of it. The tree looks something like a live-oak bonsai, only it's about five feet tall. The barbed-wire fence that the trail has been following intersects here with another that wraps up the hillside from the west. With the sounds of the crickets and small birds, this spot feels just like you're inside an Ansel Adams photograph.

Despite all of the cattle trails branching here and there, it's not hard to understand which trail is Bolinas Ridge Trail until you get to the fork at mile 3.6. Go left, continuing on Bolinas Ridge Trail, as the option to the right is just a well-used cattle trail. There are long views to the west of the green hillsides above Point Reyes National Seashore. Somewhere between you and those hills runs CA 1. In a quarter mile the trail juts up sharply again for a 50-foot rocky climb, at the top of which you can look north and sight Tomales Bay one more time.

The trail rolls along through a few more quick climbs, downhills, and technical sections before passing under a small stand of three rather large eucalyptus trees. They provide shade, and the spot beneath them is quite popular.

At mile 5 you come to yet another metal gate with chain latch. This is the last gate until you make the return trip. Past this gate some coyote brush crowds in on the trail, and the foliage in general increases, with the barbed-wire fence getting eaten up by berry vines, ferns, and other lush types of greenery. Keep an eye out for a quick downhill that features many ruts running down it. These ruts can grab your front wheel and give you a fairly squirrelly experience, and at the bottom is a sandy wash to further test your technical abilities. After this, the trail enters into the woods proper.

At mile 5.2 the trail intersects with Shafter Bridge Trail, which splits off back and to the left. Proceed straight on Bolinas Ridge Trail. Very shortly after that, a dense pine forest appears on the left-hand side of the trail, only to swallow the trail whole in the next 110 yards, like a 50-foot green pipeline.

The woods section is incredibly fun, and if it feels faster than the first half of the ride, it's because it is. Having started at an elevation of just under 400 feet, the bulk of the climbing is done within the first 5 miles, gaining almost 1,100 feet, leaving just 500 feet to gain in the last 6 miles.

The pine forest gradually turns into redwoods, and the dark, healthy soil is moist beneath your wheels, cushioned with decomposing leaves and pine needles. Although the trail is still slightly climbing through here, it feels very fast, with quick ups and downs and many slight turns. The weaving and rolling of the trail has a very energetic, almost frenetic quality, and riding it imbues one with a spirit of the woods or of the trail. You get caught up on whatever motive inspired that winding path, as though the trail is desperately searching for the perfect tree, or perhaps some trinket it lost along the way. Eventually you find yourself obsessively mashing the pedals, driving your body and machine forward as quickly as possible, and you can almost hear the voice of Gollum echoing in your head. Fortunately, the spirit never finds whatever it is searching for.

In the midst of this frantic search, there is a trail junction, at mile 6.2, where Randall Trail comes up the 1.5 miles from CA 1 on the right.

The next fork comes up at mile 8, and a half mile beyond that you emerge from the trees for the first time on an extended downhill before quickly reentering the trees and going up another kicker. Just another half mile on, you come to another exposed downhill section, but this one is different. Here the soil has turned from the coffee-colored stuff inside the woods to yellow-orange, while the flora on either side has changed to chaparral. The trail drops off in front of you, turning down the hill to the left. Over the tops of the low chaparral bushes, you can see the ocean. If you take a moment to stop, there is a short post you can carefully stand on to get a better view of Bolinas and Stinson Beach, with the thin peninsula that extends between them featuring prominently as it encapsulates Bolinas Lagoon.

Don't allow your legs to get too cold while enjoying the views of Stinson and Bolinas, though, because there's still a short way to the end of this trail. The descent continues through that left-hand turn, but then quickly turns back into a climb featuring loose rocks. There is another fork here, but it's only a Pacific Gas and Electric access road—well marked as such. You pop back into the woods for the next 2 miles, and the trail is slightly downhill through this section. Perhaps because of the lack of gradient, and also the closer proximity to the shore, it is especially moist, and the condensed water forms puddles on the trail.

The trail dead-ends at a wide metal gate, where it makes a T into Fairfax-Bolinas Road. There is a small dirt parking lot here, which is where you'll find your ride home, if you have arranged for one. If you didn't arrange for a ride, then you've got an 11-mile return trip, but fortunately it's mostly downhill.

After the Ride

The nearest low-price option for replenishing yourself after this long ride is the Olema Liquor and Deli (phone (415) 663-8615), just a mile from the trailhead down Sir Francis Drake Boulevard, where it meets CA 1. At the same intersection, you have a high-price option—the Olema Inn & Restaurant—but you'd better make reservations ahead (phone (415) 663-9559). Just a little farther north on CA 1 is Point Reyes Station and a slew of other restaurant options, including the local favorite, Pine Cone Diner (phone (415) 663-1536).

SLEEPY HOLLOW: SLEEPY HOLLOW OUT-AND-BACK

In Brief

This ride takes you out along the ridges that define the geography of northern San Rafael and back. Sneaking a peak at a few of the snazzy high-dollar homes that spice up these classic Northern California hillsides makes this basic out-and-back fire-road run something interesting. A good one to check out once, or a great workout if you live in the area.

Contact

Marin County Open Space District
Marin County Civic Center
3501 Civic Center Drive, Room 415
San Rafael, CA 94903
(415) 499-6387
District field office: (415) 499-6405
www.co.marin.ca.us/depts/PK/Main/mcosd/
os_park_30.asp

Description

Starting from the tiny dirt parking lot across from Muir Court on Lucas Valley Road, there is a wooden gate with a green sign welcoming one to Terra Linda/Sleepy Hollow Divide Open Space Preserve. Pass through the pedestrian opening in the wooden gate and head up

DIRECTIONS

From the Golden Gate Bridge, drive 16 miles north on US 101 to the Lucas Valley Road exit. Head west on Lucas Valley Road exactly 2 miles from the highway to the small dirt parking lot on the left-hand side of the road, opposite Muir Court. There is a wooden gate with Terra Linda/ Sleepy Hollow Divide Open Space Preserve signs posted on it.

Note: Because the ride starts with a very steep climb, you might consider parking closer to the freeway and riding to the actual trailhead to give the legs a warm up. Lucas Valley Road is very bike-friendly.

KEY AT-A-GLANCE INFORMATION

Length: 7.54 miles

Configuration: Out-and-back

Difficulty: 3/10; just one steep climb up onto the ridge

Scenery: Ridgeline views of the entire Lucas Valley and Mount Tamalpais

Exposure: Well-done; only a couple of shady spots, but one is perfectly placed at the top of the first climb.

Ride traffic: Minimal; only locals hit these fire roads

Riding time: 1–1.5 hours

Access: Free parking around Lucas Valley Road

Facilities: None

GPS TRAILHEAD COORDINATES (WGS 84)

UTM Zone 10S
Easting 0537180
Northing 4206600
Latitude N 38° 1' 36.4"
Longitude W 122° 34' 21.7"

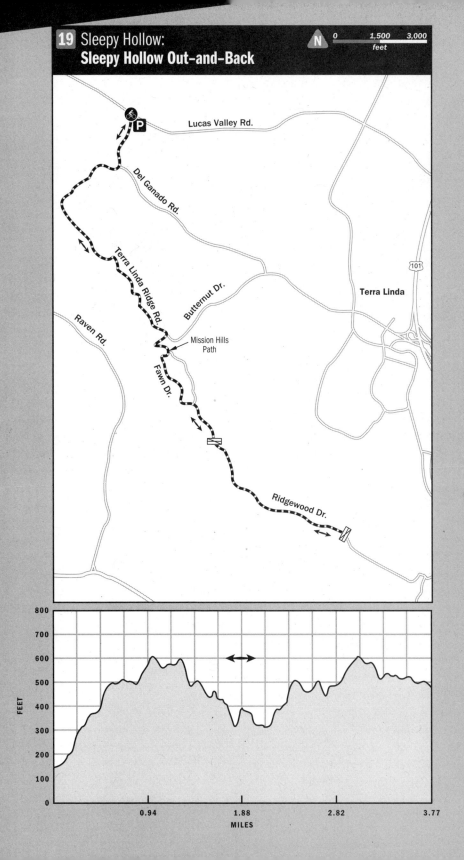

N

0   1,500   3,000
        feet

Lucas Valley Rd.

Del Ganado Rd.

Terra Linda Ridge Rd.

Butternut Dr.

Raven Rd.

Mission Hills
Path

Fawn Dr.

Terra Linda

101

Ridgewood Dr.

800
700
600
500
FEET
400
300
200
100
0

0.94   1.88   2.82   3.77
MILES

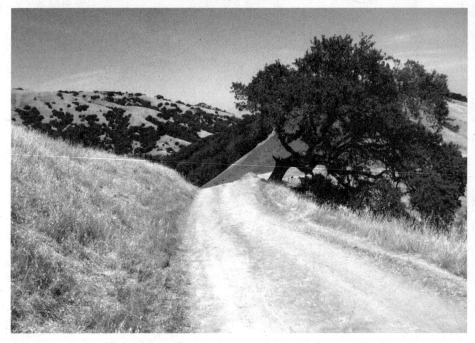

An oak beckons you to take a quick nap in the cool shade.

the fire road. The first 200 yards are basically flat, running past a rock gate house, a white corral, an old dead oak, and then into a stretch lined primarily with bay trees. It kicks up dramatically as the road passes under some oak and bay trees. But then the trees let up, and you're thrown out into the sun, with a rock-strewn grassy hillside on your left to keep you company.

The trail starts climbing seriously—feels steep, doesn't it?! The fire-road surface is not bad—no looser than your typical dirt road—but the angle you're ascending exacerbates whatever traction issues might exist, so try to stay seated to keep the weight over the rear wheel. Unfortunately, when you come to the fork, you must make the right turn up the steep switchback and continue heading up the hill. Just about now you're beginning to understand the suggestion of riding a mile or two to the trailhead to warm up your legs. Yes, because you're gaining 350 feet in elevation in just two-thirds of a mile. From this vantage point, you can see a high-tech, solar panel–bedecked home slightly obscured by the large oaks. And looking east across the valley, you can see the light blue roof of the Frank Lloyd Wright–designed Marin Civic Center nestled in front of San Pedro Mountain. The Marin Civic Center is a truly incredible building if you get an opportunity to see it up close.

Finally at about mile 1, you reach the top of the ridge, roughly 605 feet above sea level. There is a beautiful, gigantic live-oak tree and a rock that looks just like a miniature version of Half Dome to greet you at the top. They sit next to each other on the downhill edge of the trail, and the tree leans off down the hill and doesn't offer the trail any shade after about midday. This is a scenic spot to catch your breath.

After you make a left at the next fork, the trail descends for a couple hundred feet before

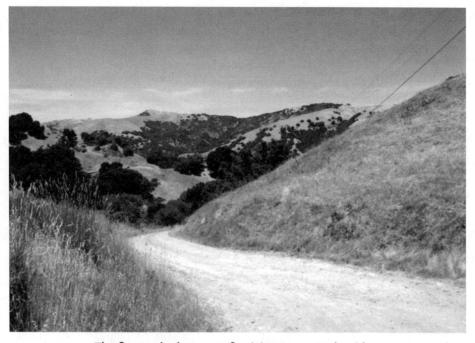

The fire road takes an unforgiving route up the ridge.

rounding a left-hand bend and hitting another steep climb. Make another left at the next fork, continuing on Terra Linda Ridge fire road, and as you crest this short climb, the view to the south opens up and you can see Mt. Tamalpais off in the distance. The trail along the top of the ridge is slightly concave, and during the rainy season water will collect in large puddles covering the whole road. There are small singletracks that have been carved in on either side of these concave spots for the purpose of avoiding these puddles when it's wet.

As you ride along this straight, exposed section, the views all around are excellent, with the hills rolling off on either side and expansive oak groves, grassy hillsides, and clusters of homes interplaying with each other to create a visual feast. After a short descent, Irving fire road appears on the right at mile 1.4, but you will continue left on Terra Linda Ridge fire road and then left again onto Terra Linda fire road when area namesake Sleepy Hollow fire road pops out at you on the right. Sleepy Hollow fire road, as well as all of the other turns off Terra Linda Ridge fire road, is just a short trail running down into the surrounding neighborhoods. There is nothing too notable about them, but they're worth doing a few out-and-backs if you've got a little more energy in your legs than the 7.5 miles of this ride call for.

The trail gradually rolls down the ridge, scrubbing about a hundred feet of elevation, and as the sight lines change, you can see a *very* nice home with a huge vanishing-edge swimming pool. Go through an S-curve and the fire road turns into a decrepit old paved path. There is a beautiful oak tree nestled in the turn here, and a low, curved brick wall. The paved path might have been a driveway at some point, and it almost seems as though the plot was once intended for a private home and the project abandoned.

The badly paved path Ts into a nicer paved path, which is Mission Hills Bike Path. Make a right and head down the sharp descent that ends in another of the wooden gates such as the one you passed through to start the ride. The pedestrian openings in these gates *are* wide enough to ride through, *just*. It would seem many have tried and failed as there are many handlebar-height nicks and scratches in the wooden posts, probably left by those who misjudged their passage. There must be some sore fingers and elbows out there.

Once through the gate, make a left turn onto Fawn Drive. This is a paved residential road, and this community is somewhat remote, so be respectful as you ride through this semiprivate, nongated community. The road climbs steadily and levels out a little when it makes a right at the point where Fox Lane connects with it. Continue right on Fawn Drive.

At mile 2.6 you will come to a gate that has some very large signs marked PRIVATE and PERMISSION CAN BE REVOKED, which are to discourage use of the road that passes through it. The fire road is tucked back in this small gated community. Basically, just mind your business through here and be respectful. Pass by the three homes and then hit the dirt again, and you're on Ridgewood fire road.

Turn left at the fork, staying on Ridgewood (right option is Tomahawk fire road). The scenery changes in here to eucalyptus forest. It is pretty but not quite as enchanting a forest as that found on the Lake Chabot ride. The fire road is noticeably rockier on Ridgewood. Make another left, and then the trail descends a little before ending at another wooden gate at Ridgewood Drive. Turn around and head back the way you came, remembering that all but the last turn on Terra Linda Ridge fire road will be right-handers in this direction.

After the Ride

There are a few food options in the Terra Linda Shopping Center. Make a right back onto Lucas Valley Road and another right onto Las Gallinas Avenue about a half mile before you reach the freeway. Head about a mile and then make a right onto Manuel T. Freitas Parkway and another right onto Del Ganado Road, and you'll see the shopping center. A favorite here is Panchitos Mexican Restaurant at 667 Del Ganado Road behind the supermarket. This is a casual dining place with unbelievably good burritos and salsa. You can get outta here, full, for about $15, depending on what you get on your burrito and whether you go for imported or domestic variety brews (phone (415) 472-6766). If you're craving pizza, try Lo Coco's on the same street (phone (415) 472-3323).

KEY AT-A-GLANCE INFORMATION

Length: 2.17 miles

Configuration: Counterclockwise loop

Difficulty: 3/10; short and flat, but slightly technical

Scenery: Rolling, oak-dotted Petaluma hills

Exposure: Medium; you won't get too cooked in this park.

Ride traffic: Generally low, but due to park's small size, moderate rushes on evenings and weekends can make the park feel crowded.

Riding time: 0.5–0.75 hours.

Access: $3 parking fee in parking lot

Facilities: Restrooms and water fountains

GPS TRAILHEAD COORDINATES (WGS 84)

UTM Zone   10S
Easting   0529554
Northing   4229226
Latitude   N 38° 12' 46.87"
Longitude   W 122° 39' 43.69"

HELEN PUTNAM REGIONAL PARK: "DON'T STOP 'TIL YOU GET ENOUGH"

In Brief

A favorite of local mountain bikers and cyclocrossers, Helen Putnam is a tiny 216-acre park hidden in the hills just outside Petaluma, in among the free-range cattle ranches, chicken and grain farms, and nice urban homes. The ride demonstrated here comprises the largest contiguous loop possible in the park, and it's still quite short at 2.17 miles. But it is so much fun, with tight turns, five-inch-wide singletrack throughout, no extended climbing, and rapidly changing scenery, that it feels like a much bigger park. This is a great loop for multiple laps—just like Michael Jackson said, "Don't stop 'til you get enough."

Contact

Helen Putnam Regional Park
411 Chileno Valley Road
Petaluma, CA 94952
(707) 433-1625 or 565-2041
www.sonoma-county.org/parks/pk_helen.htm

Description

The Native American Pomo and Miwok tribes originally inhabited the area known as Petaluma. The name is taken from a Miwok phrase meaning "hill backside," which, it is believed, references Sonoma Mountain lying on the northeast side kitty-corner across town from little Helen Putnam Regional Park.

DIRECTIONS

From the Golden Gate Bridge, drive approximately 31 miles north to Petaluma. Exit onto Petaluma Boulevard South, drive 2.5 miles through old town Petaluma, and make a left onto Western Avenue. Drive 2 miles up Western Avenue and make a left onto Chileno Valley Road. Helen Putnam Regional Park is 0.6 mile from Western Avenue on your left.

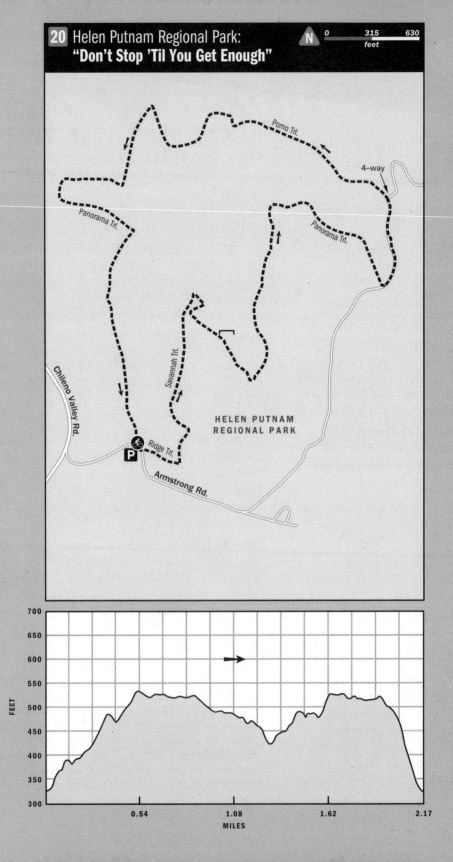

N

0   315   630
feet

Pomo Trl.

4–way

Panorama Trl.

Panorama Trl.

Savannah Trl.

Chileno Valley Rd.

HELEN PUTNAM
REGIONAL PARK

Ridge Trl.

P

Armstrong Rd.

700
650
600
550
500
450
400
350
300

FEET

0.54   1.08   1.62   2.17
MILES

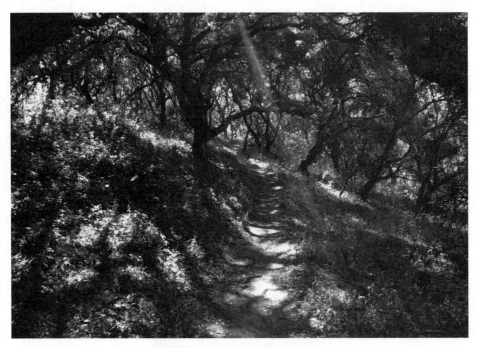

Tight singletrack in the woods

From the parking lot, head up toward the restroom but veer right and locate the trailhead sign just off the paved path. Head past the sign and through the hole in the fence onto the dirt trail that climbs steeply up the hill. This is Ridge Trail. (The paved path is also known as Ridge Trail). There is good traction on this steep climb, but a few wooden water breaks punctuate it, which adds a bit of technical aspect.

Ride for just 500 feet and then make a left onto Savannah Trail, which is an awesome, tight singletrack trail winding up through one of the wooded areas of the park. Be careful because there is a ton of poison oak on the ground—it loves the conditions provided by the moisture of the creek running through the little cut and the shade of the trees. Don't fall off, and keep in mind that riding off the trail a few inches exposes your tires to the oils of the plant and could result in skin exposure later if you should need to remove your wheels to put your bike back in/on the car.

Make a right at the next fork, which takes you around a switchback and up a steep 20-foot climb with roots and rocks. At the top it levels out, but you're still in among the trees and poison oak. As you weave your body in and out of the trees lining the trail and try to keep your tires on dirt and not on rash-inducing plants, watch for the next fork and make a right. In another 50 yards, the trees open up, and there is a bench overlooking the beautiful grassy hillsides with clusters of oak trees, but you probably won't want to stop the roller coaster.

Fifteen feet beyond the bench is another intersection. Turn left through the trees and find an even more awesome deep-woods singletrack. This is the kind of singletrack that makes you feel like Luke Skywalker or Princess Leia when they were racing the imperial

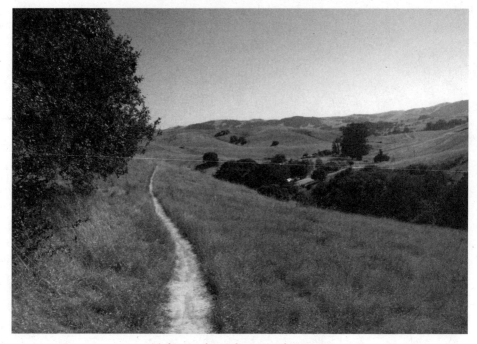

Tight singletrack out in the open

speeder bikes through the forest in *Return of the Jedi*. Or, if you're not into the whole Jedi knight thing, you might just feel like a mountain biker having a kick-ass time weaving through the trees.

Once you exit the trees, the singletrack becomes surrounded on both sides with three-foot tall grass. The trail surface through these grassy sections has a bunch of small but deep potholes, about the size of horse hooves. What these are, actually, are pits left from the removal of clumps of the tall grass from the trail, as the root structures tend to pull up a lot of dirt with them.

Make a right at the next unmarked fork in the grass and then another right at the next fork, which puts you on Panorama Trail (marked). Ride another 700 feet on a slight downhill through the tall grass and come to a five-way intersection. Here you'll make the sharpest left, about 150 degrees behind you, onto Pomo Trail, which is marked with a sign. If so desired, you could extend the ride here by crossing the paved Ridge Trail onto South Loop Trail, which is a half-mile loop with a 15-yard out-and-back, and then coming back onto Pomo Trail.

Pomo Trail parallels paved Ridge Trail for a few yards before diving back into the woods. Go straight through the four-way intersection, staying on Pomo, which offers up another generous helping of amazing singletrack!

Make two consecutive lefts, continuing on Pomo Trail, and enter into one of the best sections of the trail as it cuts sharp turns through the woods, featuring a couple of short climbs and descents. There are some water-control boards running across the trail through here, but they are easy to ride over. In the late afternoon, the sun will shine through the trees in well-defined beams, lighting up various sections of the forest floor into an incredible mosaic of color.

At the next four-way intersection, turn right onto Panorama Trail. This is a great little downhill add-on, which winds right along the hillside and cuts a sharp left down the hill. I say add-on, because going left will actually take you to where this little loop does, just about a quarter mile sooner. This is one of the steeper sections in the park and also the roughest, with a bunch of those small grass-clump potholes mentioned earlier chewing up the trail surface.

Turn right at the intersection of Pomo Trail (L) and Panorama Trail (R) and right again at the next fork. This is the other steep section in the park. The trail goes straight down the face of the hill and has been widened a lot, presumably due to the steepness and people's lack of control going through here. Just hang over the back of the saddle and go for it. As an added pleasure, there are humongous water control beams running across the trail right at the steepest parts. There are three of these six-foot-long beams in succession, and they are fairly tall—roughly six to eight inches above the trail surface. It's sketchy to jump things on a decline this steep, but if you're talented, go for it. Otherwise, it's possible to ride around the side: the most well-worn line is around the left side, but even this isn't carefree, because there are deep potholes at each end.

From here the parking lot is in sight, but even though the trail levels out, you'll have to contend with three more of those beams to get back to base. And then . . . head back out for another loop—or eight.

After the Ride

Eat at Old Chicago Pizza. Simple as that. Everything about this restaurant is great, from the atmosphere to the pizza itself. The building that the restaurant is located in has a storied history, and old downtown Petaluma was featured in the film *American Graffiti*. To get there, just get back on Western Avenue and head down to Petaluma Boulevard. Old Chicago Pizza is at 41 North Petaluma Boulevard, right at the junction with Western Avenue. Perfect (phone (707) 763-3897).

KEY AT-A-GLANCE INFORMATION

Length: 8.45 miles

Configuration: Double-helix, ink-blot, tangled rope . . .

Difficulty: 8/10; not a lot of climbing to be had in this small park, but it does receive high ranking in the technicality department

Scenery: Trails, trails everywhere: you see a trail and you can ride it.

Exposure: Medium

Ride traffic: High; this is one of *the* places to mountain bike in the North Bay, so the park is crawling with mountain bikers.

Riding time: 1.75–2.25 hours

Access: $2 day-use fee; 6-month passes also available

Facilities: None

GPS TRAILHEAD COORDINATES (WGS 84)

UTM Zone 10S
Easting 0575990
Northing 4233530
Latitude N 38° 14' 54.3"
Longitude W 122° 7' 53.7"

ROCKVILLE HILLS REGIONAL PARK: THE BLACK MAP

In Brief

Rockville is, as the name implies, rocky. It is also one of the top rider's parks in the Bay Area (a full-access, condensed bundle of mountain biking joy)—like a skate park, but for 26-inch wheeled, fully suspended aluminum trail rovers. If you love ultratechnical singletrack, aren't necessarily the fittest (that is, don't like to climb so much), and enjoy nature with a chance of walking out, this is the ideal park for you. North Bay mountain bikers are lucky to have the Rockville–Annadel–Skyline trifecta in such close proximity.

Contact

Rockville Hills Regional Park
2110 Rockville Road
Fairfield, CA 94534
(707) 249-3613
www.ci.fairfield.ca.us/cs-rockvillehillspark.htm

Description

When Frank Zappa wrote his song "The Black Page," he crafted such a technical, difficult-to-perform cluster of notes that the sheet music was said to look like a "black page." This ride is named "The Black Map" in honor of that song, as the topographical map is similarly dense with things to play, although in this case those things are trails, not notes. This small, 630-acre park is covered in

DIRECTIONS

From San Francisco, take the Bay Bridge out of the city and head east on Interstate 80 toward Sacramento. Approximately 40 miles from the Bay Bridge, exit I-80 onto Suisun Valley Road. Make a left, passing under the freeway, to head north on Suisun Valley Road for 1.7 miles. Make a left onto Rockville Road and drive 0.75 miles; look for the parking lot on the left.

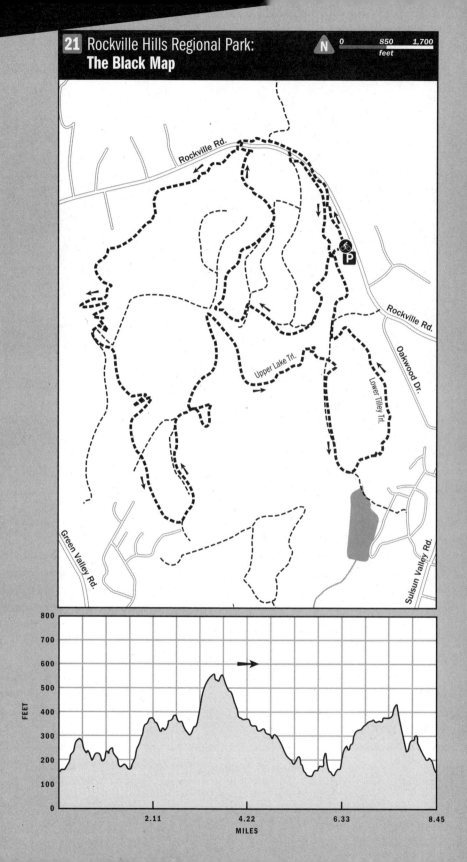

N

0   850   1,700
feet

Rockville Rd.

Rockville Rd.

Oakwood Dr.

Upper Lake Trl.

Lower Tilley Trl.

Green Valley Rd.

Suisun Valley Rd.

FEET

800
700
600
500
400
300
200
100
0

2.11   4.22   6.33   8.45
MILES

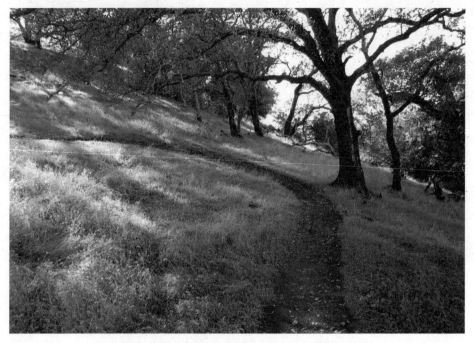

Rockville Hills Regional Park is replete with amazing singletrack turns just like this one.

trails, and every trail you see, be it fire road, doubletrack, or singletrack, you can ride. Much like in Napa's Skyline Park, another top Bay Area park for mountain bike access, you pay to play, but it is so worth it.

From the parking lot you'll notice a lot of riders heading straight up Rockville Trail, the main fire-road drag that leads straight up the hill to the lakes and the myriad of fun downhill options leading away from the lakes in all directions.

Today's ride takes a much more circuitous route up to the lakes. Head right (north) out of the parking lot, past the picnic bench, on the small singletrack that threads through a bunch of very young oak trees. This is Trail #22, or Quarry Trail, if you're not into the numbers-instead-of-names thing. It's easiest to memorize the trails in terms of the numbers, though, since that's the way they are marked throughout the park, using simple, brown plastic road markers with numbered stickers. Trail names are only given on a key on the downloadable map, and on one central signboard by the lakes.

Trail #22 is a singletrack that runs parallel to Rockville Road, just a fence and a gully away. Very quickly you get a taste of the rocks that influenced this park's name, of the reddish, lava type. Throughout the park, trail surface is either sticky, clay-based dirt, or gnarly rock.

Not far from the parking lot you come to Mini White Moab (MWM), a short section of hillside, about the size of a slanted soccer field, which has been completely cemented over, rocks and all. It really takes the concept of wall riding to a whole new level. Beyond MWM you'll find the Playground, an area of rolling terrain with trails cutting between nearly every manzanita bush. At the center of this little dirt playground is a nine-foot-tall rock spire; be careful because there tends to be a great deal of broken beer bottles surrounding this rock formation.

Beyond the Playground the chaparral really takes over, and you find yourself contorting every which way to squeeze through the low manzanita bushes and around the boulders. This isn't the speediest section of trail in the world, but it's fun, like a game of Twister.

The methodology for the first 3 miles of this ride is to go right. Go right at every intersection, marked and (often) unmarked, following the fence line as it wraps around to the west, harnessing in this spirited park. The first three-quarter-mile section of park is very hectic, with MWM, an odd paved section (Trail #23, Old Ranch Road), technical boulder sections, random trails intersecting every 30 yards, and car noises filtering in from Rockville Road. As you get to the northernmost area of the park, though, and are gradually redirected to head west, you get to see a much different aspect of the park.

This northern part is very scenic and calm compared to the rest of the park. At this point you should be on Trail #14, Unknown Trail. A low rock wall bounds this end of the park, and the trail runs along the oak-studded base of the hills of Rockville, with a large grass field extending out to the north. In late spring, a bright green sea of grass burns beneath the dark green lumps of live-oak tree clusters, and a narrow trail jets off in front of you, meandering through the trees and rocks. This is a speedy section of trail, and one that you will not be able to get enough of; it's like instant runner's high.

Continue making right turns, keeping the perimeter fence in sight as you go, and eventually the trail dives left into a cove of sorts. The first climb, a 250-footer, zigzags its way up the wall of the cove—tight singletrack clawing over exposed roots and boulder clusters, ricocheting off young trees. Tight, tight switchbacks of the type that need wood-and-post reinforcement characterize the top of the climb. These are exceedingly difficult to clear without putting a foot down, in either the uphill or downhill direction—a great challenge.

As you crest the lip of the cove, you find yourself at a crossroads on the edge of a hilltop meadow. There is a forest of adolescent oak trees up here, and if you look back off the edge of the cove you get a beautiful view across the small valley, the floor of which is cultivated fields, to a northern hill. This is the most scenic spot of the entire ride, but there is a lot more riding yet.

Make a right turn at the unmarked intersection and continue along through #12, Jockey Junction (farthest right turn), and eventually make a right onto Trail #8, Lower Mystic Trail. Tight singletrack makes its way along the western side of the hill, and at the 3-mile mark you'll climb slightly up and come to a junction with the Oakridge Drive Entrance Trail, demarked by an informative trail sign. Here you will make a left.

The trail wraps around the point of the small ridge and begins climbing up the eastern side. This is the toughest climb of the whole day, up a doubletrack that can be pretty rutted and sandy. Once on top of the ridge, you'll continue climbing for another 100 yards through the trees, and then you'll find yourself on the open ridgetop with 360-degree views. You can explore a bit up here, even opting to ride the small loop around the electrical towers, but then head down the fire road on the north side of the towers.

The fire road descends quickly down to the lakes. Ignore the early trail that splits off to the left and ride straight through the first four-way intersection to the major junction at the bottom of the hill. As you descend, you can see Lower Lake off to the right as you descend. At the major junction, go right toward Lower Lake.

Follow the fire road across a wide valley to where it splits up at the edge of a large housing development. Choose the singletrack that rides along the nearest backyard fence. This is Trail #5, Lower Lake Loop, and one of the most technical sections in the park. Strewn with rocks and roots, it descends lightly down to a small stream, which is crossed over a flattened log. You then climb up to a paved road; this is the other end of Trail #23, Old Ranch Road. Ride up this, through some elaborate fencing, and make a right turn onto Trail #3, Upper Tilley Trail. It descends for 0.25 miles to a gate labeled "Interpretive Trail." Pass through the gate.

In this southeastern leg of the park, you'll follow the same "right turns only" rule as at the beginning of the ride. The objective is to make as wide a loop as possible around this little chaparral-covered hill; however, the trails in this area can get confused with the deer trails, so the secondary goal would be to just explore. You can't get lost, since the park is completely fenced in and surrounded by houses to boot. In fact, there are a few areas where you'll be literally covered in foliage, only to pop into an open area, just 40 yards on the hill above somebody mowing their back lawn. Eventually, you should wind up in the gloamy oak woodland on the eastern side of the hill. At the north end of that, you'll make a right onto Trail #25, Devil's Backbone, which will take you back to the parking lot and prep you for the final phase of the ride.

The final phase, if you are so inclined, takes you up the main drag, Rockville Trail, up to the lakes. Follow it all the way to Upper Lake, which you'll now have an opportunity to explore. Ride clockwise around the lake and pass through the gate on the other side, depositing yourself onto Trail #18, Rock Gardens. Climb up and follow this out along the ridge. There are a lot of trails that peel off to the left; continue to the right, because you're looking for the ultimate: Trail #20, Cave Trail, which is a steep, waterfall dive down the hill. Do not attempt this descent if you are prone to endos and broken clavicles: massive bike skills are required. This will drop you down to territory familiar from the beginning of the ride. Make a right and head back east. To mix it up, instead of taking Quarry Trail (#20), take Upper Quarry Trail (#21) back along the hill to the parking lot, an equally fun singletrack that actually skirts along the top of Mini White Moab.

After the Ride

Hop in the car and head back down Suisun Valley Road. Just before you get to I-80, make a right onto Mangels Boulevard and then an immediate left onto Business Center Drive. At 5055 Business Center Drive in Fairfield you'll find Pelayo's Mexican Restaurant. Slightly more expensive than your average taqueria, but you can't beat the quality or the proximity (phone (707) 863-0225).

KEY AT-A-GLANCE INFORMATION

Length: 7.86 most excellent miles

Configuration: Counterclockwise loop

Difficulty: 9/10. If it was 2 miles longer, it would get a full 10.

Scenery: Gorgeous rock-garden-encrusted, mountain-bike-legal singletrack rolling through classic Napa County oak forest.

Exposure: Medium-rare

Ride traffic: Very popular on the weekends

Riding time: 2–3 hours

Access: $4 just to ride your bike in, $6 to drive in. Park closes 1 hour before sunset; your car will be locked in if you're not out in time. Trails are closed 5 days following rain; call ahead for current conditions.

Facilities: Water, restrooms, campground, disc golf course!

GPS TRAILHEAD COORDINATES (WGS 84)

UTM Zone 10S
Easting 0565700
Northing 4236860
Latitude N 38° 16' 45.4"
Longitude W 122° 14' 55.8"

SKYLINE WILDERNESS PARK: SINGLESPEEDER'S DELIGHT

In Brief

Perhaps all that needs to be said about this park is that it is going to be the site of the 2008 Singlespeed World Championships (SSWC; **www.sswc08.com**). Never mind that it has hosted World Cup Mountain Bike Races, numerous local mountain bike races, and is just a very well-run park in a beautiful location with phenomenal access for mountain bikers. Skyline Wilderness Park rates in the top five Bay Area mountain biking destinations, and you definitely don't have to be a singlespeeder to enjoy it.

Contact

Skyline Wilderness Park
2201 Imola Avenue
Napa, CA 94559
(707) 252-0481
www.ncfaa.com/skyline/skyline_park.htm

Description

When I revisited Skyline Park for the purposes of the book, after a seven-year hiatus, I decided to take my singlespeed cyclocross bike, since I had been gradually falling in love with the quiet simplicity of the thing and thought that it would be a nice approach for the technical singletrack I remembered from the park. I also knew that the 2008

DIRECTIONS

From San Francisco, head east across the Bay Bridge, take Interstate 80 north 30 miles through Vallejo, and take Exit 33 to CA 37 West/Marine World Parkway. Drive 2 miles on CA 37 West, take Exit 19 to CA 29 North toward Napa, and drive 7.2 miles. Follow the merge from CA 29/CA 12 onto Napa Vallejo Highway, drive 2.6 miles, and turn right onto Imola Avenue. Skyline Wilderness Park is located 1 mile up Imola Avenue on the right just before the road's first major left turn.

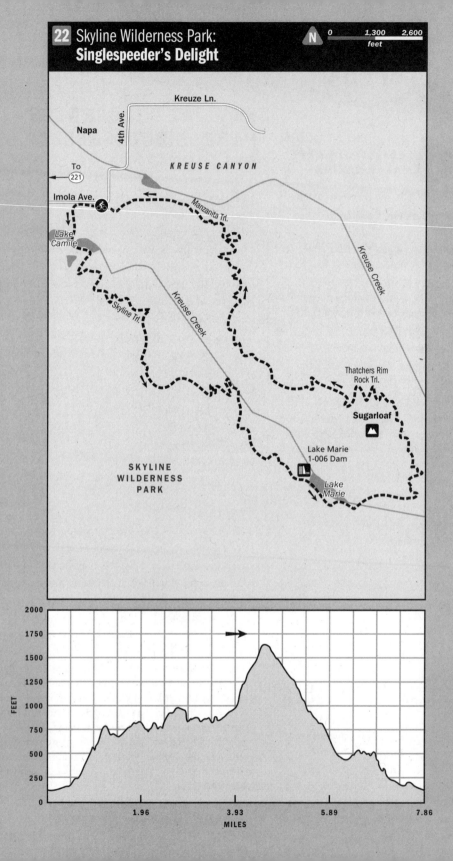

N

0   1,300   2,600
feet

Kreuze Ln.

Napa

4th Ave.

KREUSE CANYON

To
221

Imola Ave.

Manzanita Trl.

Kreuse Creek

Lake
Camile

Skyline Trl.

Kreuse Creek

Thatchers Rim
Rock Trl.

Sugarloaf

**SKYLINE
WILDERNESS
PARK**

Lake Marie
1-006 Dam

Lake
Marie

2000
1750
1500
1250
1000
750
500
250
0

FEET

1.96   3.93   5.89   7.86
MILES

Singlespeed World Championships would be taking place in the park, and since I fully intend on competing (if I am lucky enough to get a spot), I knew that it would be great preparation to ride the machine that I would be racing. I opted to do the largest loop around the perimeter of the park and also tackle Thatchers Rim Rock Trail, which I had never ridden. The ride and the bike were a perfect match, and I rode the whole thing in a dream state.

One of the aspects that makes this park different from other parks is the fee system. You don't get into this park for free; whether you walk in, ride in, or drive in with a horse trailer, you're going to pay something. It's $6 to drive a car in with a mountain bike, and a whopping $4 per person to bike in, but it is entirely worth it, as this park has some of the most progressive stances on mountain bike access in all of the Bay Area. The park is run by a private nonprofit organization, and the good quality of the facilities and trails speaks volumes about the management.

After paying your entrance fee, head to the northwest side of the parking lot, find the graveled Lake Marie Road, and follow that as it wraps left around the stables. Watch on your right for the sign leading to Skyline Trail. You'll ride through the 220-yard, chain link fence–lined "Corridor," which is designed to protect the Lake Camille wildlife restoration area and has a speed limit of 5 mph.

Upon exiting the Corridor make a right toward Skyline/Buckeye, indicated by a hand-painted sign. In the first 55 yards, you pass Buckeye Trail on the left and River to Ridge Trail on the right, after which you are faced with a choice between Skyline Trail and Lower Skyline Trail. Both are incredible singletracks that lead to the same place, but where Skyline Trail clambers up the largely treeless, rocky hillside, Lower Skyline Trail takes a slightly smoother and stealthier route through the trees. Regardless which option you take, your singletrack jones will be fulfilled within just a few yards of trail, and your brain will fill with dopamine while your body settles into a rhythm of balancing contortions and carefully modulated outburst of power.

The next intersection is the reunification of the Skyline Trail siblings; proceed in a southbound direction on Skyline Trail (not lower), which is thankfully marked by a sign. It's a twisty singletrack descent 0.25 miles to the next junction with Bayleaf Trail. The general rule for the rest of the ride to Lake Marie is to make all right-hand turns, staying on Skyline Trail.

What follows for the next 2.2 miles is some of the greatest rolling terrain singletrack ever devised. The trail gods created this trail expressly for a 29-inch-wheeled bike with a 32/14 ratio—the ups and downs are all very quick and mild, allowing the rider to keep up a constant speed with measured bursts of pedaling, careful pumping of the arms, and skilled, minimalist use of brakes. The reddish brown line of the trail cutting through oak trees and the yellowish green grass draw you along with a determined breath, like a greyhound chasing the lure. The taut chain doesn't slap and the only sound over the frequent rock gardens is the subtle chaffing of high-pressure rubber tires grappling with rocks for traction.

At mile 2.4 you come to another junction with Buckeye Trail, at which you make the requisite right turn to stay on Skyline Trail, but here there are six log steps leading up the first 30 yards of trail. These steps are tricky but doable. You enter a wooded section, make a right at the next junction, and pass by a brick chimney and crumbled foundation of an old house. Beyond this you can begin to see Lake Marie glimmering up at you through the woods.

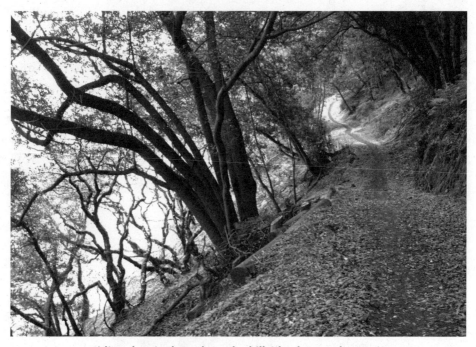

Riding the singletrack on the hillside above Lake Marie

The next intersection you come to is Chaparral Trail, and if you are at all averse to hike-a-biking, you should turn left here and avoid Thatchers Rim Rock Trail up ahead. Chaparral Trail is a challenging singletrack that runs down Marie Creek, replete with slick boulder drops, exposed roots, and the delicious smell of decomposing biomatter. It's an excellent option to hauling self and equipment up over Sugarloaf Peak.

For those of you prepared for a unique challenge, continue on Skyline Trail about 0.5 miles past Chaparral Trail and make a left onto Thatchers Rim Rock Trail. This ride is called Singlespeeder's Delight not just for the momentum magic of Skyline Trail, but also for this wall climb up the backside of Sugarloaf Peak. Why? Lighter bike = easier portage. Very little about the tight, steep switchbacks up the south face of the mountain can be ridden in either direction, so be prepared to shoulder your bike all the way up the average 20 percent gradient to the top. But the descent down the north face of the mountain will more than make up for time spent hoofing.

Sugarloaf Peak itself is a special place, with both commanding views and cozy, squat live oaks, but it's the descent down that will command a special place in your heart forever after. Much like an open-air/chaparral version of the Whittemore Gulch descent through the redwoods in the South Bay's Purisima Creek, this trail zigzags down through tight switchbacks that almost demand the ability to commit controlled endo-tail-flicks as you float down 1,200 feet in 1.8 miles of uninterrupted trail.

At the bottom make a left to avoid hikers-only Marie Creek Trail and then turn right onto Manzanita Trail about 45 yards past that. Here again, as with the trip up Skyline Trail,

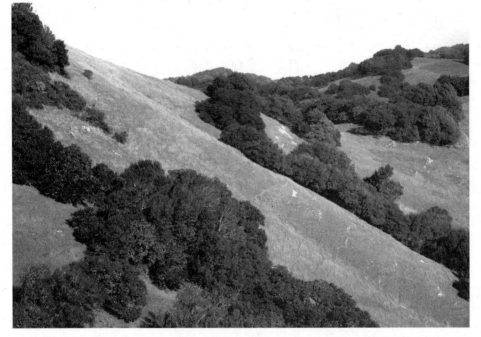

View from the hike-a-bike up Thatchers Rim Rock Trail

make a series of right turns in order to stay on the outermost trail, Manzanita Trail. The soil on the east side of Marie Creek is sandier, following suit with the chaparral ecosystem. Keep an eye on your speedometer, because at 6.7 miles Manzanita Trail splits, and the left half is hikers-only (this wasn't well marked in this direction). The mountain bike bypass is wildly technical, with one particular 22-yard boulder section that is destined to topple the unwary. The descent down Manzanita Trail is full of surprises, including a few random water bars, so keep those arms bent at the ready until you cross the bridge and enter the disc golf course. From there just get on the gravel road and spin your 32/14 on back to the parking lot.

After the Ride

Napa being what Napa is—a wine country resort town—it's tough to find good and cheap nonchain food. But there are a few fun options in town: Big D Burgers (phone (707) 255-7188) at 1005 Silverado Trail (turn right from Imola Avenue onto Soscol Avenue and drive 1.4 miles north, merging onto Silverado Trail), a locally owned burger joint; Old Adobe Bar & Grill (phone (707) 255-4310) at 376 Soscol Avenue (half mile north of Imola Avenue), a dive bar/nightclub that masquerades as a restaurant with great atmosphere; and El Potrillo Mexican Food (phone (707) 257-6925) at 640 Third Street (drive 1.3 miles north on Soscol Avenue, turn right on Third Street). Then again, if you're vacationing in Napa, you're probably prepared to spend some money on a few of the incredible fine-dining restaurants Napa is known for.

23

Length: 6.16 miles

Configuration: Loop with 0.2-mile out-and-back

Difficulty: 8/10. Whether you do the loop clockwise or counter-clockwise, Rough Go ensures a good physical and mental workout.

Scenery: Set in the Valley of the Moon, a setting often used in author Jack London's stories, Annadel features a wide array of landscapes, from pine forests to chaparral.

Exposure: Shade over most of the ride, with Rough Go receiving the least amount, and the area around Lake Ilsanjo receiving the most.

Ride traffic: Heavy on weekends, moderate on weekday afternoons and evenings

Riding time: 0.75–1.25 hours

Access: There is a fee to park beyond the ranger station, and it varies with season: Memorial Day– Labor Day, $6; rest of the year, $5. It is feasible to park off-site and ride into the park. The park is open from sunrise to sunset.

Facilities: There are restrooms and water fountains in the parking lot. During summer there is a concession stand within riding distance to the north of the parking lot on the bank of Spring Lake. Midway through the ride, at Lake Ilsanjo, there is an outhouse-style restroom.

ANNADEL STATE PARK: CANYON TRAIL AND ROUGH GO LOOP

In Brief

This loop is classic Jekyll and Hyde, with Rough Go being the technical, rutted, and boulder-strewn single-track counterpoint to Canyon Trail's moderately smooth fire-road serenity. This ride is great in either direction and provides a very different experience, depending on whether you choose to climb or descend Rough Go. There is no easy spinning on Rough Go; "taking it easy" on this trail means that one of the boulder outcroppings has decided to take possession of your forward motion. However, stopping just gives you reason to take in the rolling grasslands, reddish-brown boulders, and scattered old-growth oaks.

Contact

Annadel State Park
6201 Channel Drive
Santa Rosa, CA 95409
(707) 539-3911
www.parks.ca.gov/?page_id=480

DIRECTIONS

From the Golden Gate Bridge, go 48 miles north on US 101 to CA 12 in Santa Rosa. Exit onto CA 12 east toward Sonoma and proceed 1.3 miles until it terminates at a stoplight. Continue straight through the stoplight; this will take you onto Hoen Avenue, and you will drive 1.2 miles, through the major intersections of Yulupa Avenue and Summerfield Road. After crossing Summerfield Road, make a left at the first stop sign onto Newanga Avenue. Follow Newanga Avenue (it makes a sharp right within the first 300 feet) for 0.6 miles through a nice residential area to the ranger station at the park gate. Once inside the park, follow the signs to the Oak Knolls Picnic Area. The trailhead is in the southeast corner of the parking lot and is marked with a yellow metal gate.

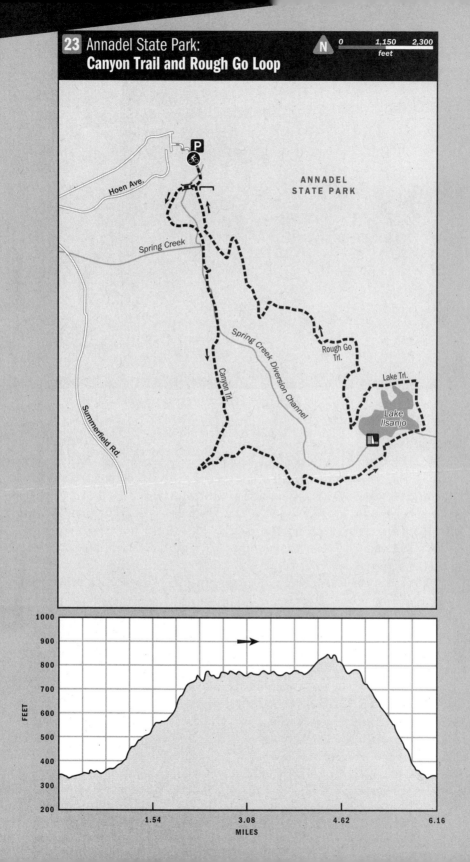

ANNADEL
STATE PARK

Hoen Ave.

Spring Creek

Spring Creek Diversion Channel

Rough Go
Trl.

Canyon Trl.

Summerfield Rd.

Lake Trl.

Lake
Ilsanjo

N

0   1,150   2,300
feet

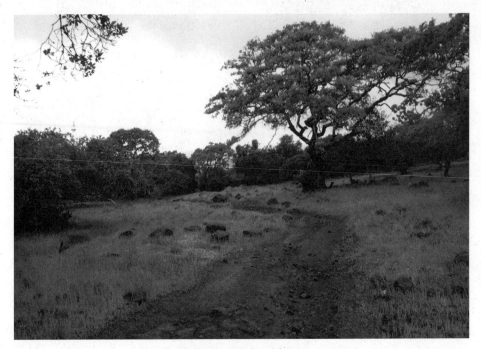

Rough Go Trail, with boulders to spare

Description

From the yellow gate in the parking lot, head right onto the unnamed gravel access road that runs along the parking lot. Look for Spring Creek to your left as you start out, and after 0.5 miles cross to the other side over an old wooden auto bridge. After the bridge continue on the gravel road and test your legs on a short, sharp, rocky climb that ascends 150 yards to the left of a large cement culvert. The trail that crosses the culvert to join the gravel road is simply another access point and only leads into a local neighborhood; you'll continue straight on the gravel road for another 0.25 miles before you come to the first major fork.

When you reach the fork, bear right or take advantage of a bench here to rest or make adjustments to your bike. Take care, as there is an abundance of poison oak growing in the creek and on the hillsides. The left option at this fork is Spring Creek Trail—another great singletrack that cuts a more direct and technical route up to man-made Lake Ilsanjo. You will definitely want to explore this trail on another ride. Today, however, take a right, crossing a second, smaller wooden bridge onto Canyon Trail.

Canyon Trail is a fire road that is alternatively smooth and choppy along its 2.6-mile length, with the choppy sections characterized by their smatterings of small, fixed "baby's head" boulders. There are a multitude of lines to take, but there is an obvious favorite line, which changes slightly after each wet season. Being one of the smoother and wider trails in the park, downhill speeds can be very fast. If you opt to ride down Canyon Trail, control your speed, give plenty of room to equestrians and hikers, and give ample vocal warnings if approaching from behind.

The climbing begins virtually from the start of the trail and continues for 1.3 miles. Ascend a mild gradient for the first 0.75 miles to the first switchback, where it kicks up slightly. The trail flattens and narrows briefly where it crosses a dry streambed, and then ramps up slightly for a 200-yard straightaway to the top of the hill. To eliminate excessive boulders in the path, this fully exposed section was completely rebuilt around the year 2000. Look for a large live oak that marks the summit of this climb, and enjoy some of the best panoramic views of Santa Rosa and the surrounding mountains on a clear day. From here the trail descends slightly and makes a sharp left before reaching the next fork.

At this fork continue straight on Canyon Trail, but note the other option—Marsh Trail, to the right, which opens up the whole back end of the park. Descend on Canyon Trail for 0.5 miles, passing a small stream and accompanying horse trough, before you come to what seems to be the termination of Canyon Trail at a T intersection on the shore of Lake Ilsanjo, which is visible through the trees. Continue following Canyon Trail to the right for another 0.6 miles around the east side of this small lake. On this east side of the lake you will find a small picnic area and an outhouse-style restroom.

As you're coming up to the next intersection of trails, the dense tree cover surrounding the lake opens up to an expansive grassy meadow, spotted with oaks. At the Lake Ilsanjo sign, make a left off Canyon Trail onto Lake Trail, an easy doubletrack that you will ride for 0.4 miles before making a right onto the aptly named Rough Go Trail. For a nice diversion, you can continue on Lake Trail another 0.1 mile as it wraps around the lake and takes you to the dam on the west side of the lake. It's a popular spot for fishing, swimming, or just relaxing. After you're done at the lake, just double-back and turn onto Rough Go Trail—there's only one way to go, since Rough Go Trail abuts into Lake Trail.

Boulders and the ruts between them define 2-mile Rough Go Trail. There *are* smooth sections of this trail, but they're too short to notice. If you're familiar with video games, this trail makes you feel like the marble in Marble Madness. Basically you'd better bring along your bike-handling credentials—or at least as much suspension travel as you can muster— and be prepared to pick through or vault your way over many of these boulder outcroppings. In many of the stickier situations, riders have carved easier alternate routes to the right or left, but it's often difficult to scan ahead and assess which is the easier choice.

From the turn off Lake Trail, Rough Go Trail begins with a 0.3-mile climb through the trees before it levels out for another 100 yards, approaching False Lake Meadow and a fork where Live Oak Trail splits off to the right. This is the first of three successive forks where you will take the left option to continue on Rough Go Trail. Past the first fork, the trail descends for a quarter mile and then levels for another quarter mile as it passes Orchard Trail on the right. Another 100 yards and the descent begins in earnest. At one point in the late 1990s, some maintenance was performed on Rough Go Trail in an attempt to make it a little less rough, and you can see the many boulders pulled from the trail on the sides of the trail. Fortunately, there were more boulders where those came from, and in just a couple seasons, Rough Go Trail restored itself to its natural difficulty, thereby avoiding having its name changed to Sorta Rough Go, or something like that.

Just 0.2 miles from the second fork comes the third at Cobblestone Trail. It's a sharp left here that leads directly into one of the more-technical 80 yards of the trail. From the

Cobblestone Trail fork it's 0.9 miles of singletrack descending and three switchbacks. Be careful descending through the boulder clusters here, which can grab your front wheel and endo your bad self all over the surrounding boulders. Success means completing the descent without putting a foot down, which requires superb pitching of body weight as well as use of controlled endo and wheelie techniques. Not ideal for speedy descents, the boulders also become quite slick when wet, which drastically alters your ability to control the bike.

Near the bottom, reach another fork and bear right. Technically this is the end of Rough Go Trail; going left will take you down to the first bridge you crossed at the beginning of the ride. For a little extra fun, though, continue to the right, passing between a fence and a large live oak. Veer to the left after the fence and follow the trail to Spring Creek. The creek bed is about 12 feet below the trail, and for most of the year, the creek is just a trickle. Try dropping into the creek bed and cranking up the steep and rocky wall on the other side. Once across, make a right turn onto the gravel access road from the start of the ride and head back to the yellow gate and the parking lot, where your hands might be too sore to operate the car keys after all the braking and gripping you did coming down Rough Go Trail.

Annadel has more than 40 miles of beautiful trails, and the Canyon Trail and Rough Go Loop are a good primer to indicate all that the park has to offer.

After the Ride

There is an abundance of great food-and-beer spots in Santa Rosa. Two great sit-down options are just across the street from the park: East West Café (phone (707) 546-6142) and Mary's Pizza Shack (phone (707) 538-1888), which are on Summerfield Road just north of Hoen Avenue. Or for a great burrito and beer, a perennial favorite among local mountain bikers is Lepe's Taqueria (phone (707) 538-8991), which you can find just a little farther north, on Montgomery Boulevard (make a right off Summerfield Road). For parts and repairs, Santa Rosa Cyclery (see appendix for contact information) is right next door to Lepe's.

**GPS TRAILHEAD
COORDINATES (WGS 84)**
UTM Zone   10S
Easting   0530740
Northing   4255220
Latitude   N 38° 26' 48.0"
Longitude   W 122° 38' 55.7"

KEY AT-A-GLANCE INFORMATION

Length: 11.95 miles

Configuration: Loop with a 0.9-mile out-and-back

Difficulty: 8/10. One more extended climb would push this ride into the 10/10 range; plenty of technical singletrack and just enough climbing.

Scenery: Natural marsh and a beautiful state park in transition

Exposure: Medium; plenty of tree cover, but loop length can result in high exposure

Ride traffic: Medium-heavy

Riding time: 2.25–3.25 hours

Access: Free parking on Channel Drive; $5 parking in the Annadel parking lot at the termination of Channel Drive

Facilities: Restrooms and water fountain at trailhead

GPS TRAILHEAD COORDINATES (WGS 84)

UTM Zone 10S
Easting 0533594
Northing 4255039
Latitude N 38° 26' 41.63"
Longitude W 122° 36' 54.04"

ANNADEL STATE PARK: WARREN RICHARDSON–NORTH BURMA LOOP

In Brief

This is the big-daddy loop in Annadel, which goes up and around the Ledson Marsh. Two Quarry Trail is one of the more challenging rides in the park, and Ridge Trail is a true gem born of the new school of trail building that has arisen in the past ten years. It's a long ride, but you'll be enjoying yourself so much you won't realize you're tired until you're back in the car.

Description

Many park users, except the equestrian crowd, park their vehicles in the dirt lot off Channel Drive when accessing the park from the northwest side. There are trails that begin just across the road from this lot, but today you'll ride 1.5 miles farther up Channel Drive to the equestrian parking lot and start the ride on Warren Richardson Trail. A trail sign with a blown-up trail map and some environmental warnings is there, as well as a drinking fountain.

Warren Richardson begins at the base of the mountain, in a shady grove of pine and bay trees and poison oak. A large gate separates you from your dream ride. Fortunately, there is an opening for pedestrian and bicycle access on the left. Pass through and begin climbing up the fire road.

DIRECTIONS

From the Golden Gate Bridge, drive approximately 49 miles north on Highway CA 101 to Santa Rosa. Exit onto CA 12 east toward Sonoma and drive 1.5 miles to Farmers Lane. Turn left on Farmers Lane and drive 0.8 miles to Montgomery Drive. Turn right and take Montgomery Drive 2.7 miles to Channel Drive. Turn right onto Channel Drive and drive 0.75 miles to the dirt parking lot on the left side of the road. From here it is a pleasant 1.5-mile ride farther down Channel Drive to the trailhead.

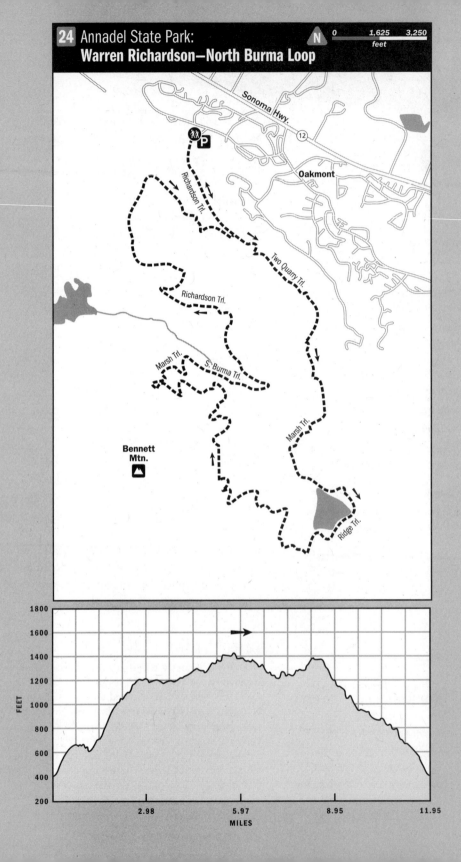

N

0   1,625   3,250
feet

Sonoma Hwy.

12

Oakmont

Richardson Trl.

Two Quarry Trl.

Richardson Trl.

Marsh Trl.

S. Burma Trl.

Bennett
Mtn.

Marsh Trl.

Ridge Trl.

1800
1600
1400
1200
1000
800
600
400
200

FEET

2.98   5.97   8.95   11.95

MILES

The ride begins with a 4-percent-grade climb up through the primarily pine forest mixed with oaks, live oaks, madrones, and some maple trees. The trail surface is gravel, with some minor ruts running here and there. In just under a mile you'll come to a small clearing that features a right-hand switchback with a picnic bench and a park sign. At the apex of the turn, Two Quarry Trail peels off left and disappears into the woods, which are somewhat dark and foreboding at this junction due to the way the ridge blocks the sun. Head into the darkness that is Two Quarry Trail.

Two Quarry is a singletrack, and the technical aspect of the trail presents itself immediately with a sharp left-hand switchback that cuts across one of the rocky seasonal streams. This type of switchback is typical in Annadel, though each one is a little different from the next. The level of technicality depends on the rock formation that the winter waters have revealed by washing away the dirt.

Despite its dark entrance, Two Quarry quickly brightens up as the pine trees begin to give way to more-low-lying maple and buckeye trees. The middle of this trail is the most difficult, as the dirt gives way to a primarily blue shale rock and the climb kicks up to an average 8 percent grade. You might find yourself having to put a foot down often, unless you have impeccable bike-handling skills. This trail used to be even rockier, to the point where it was nearly impossible to climb, because the rocks were inches deep, like monstrous gravel, and afforded little in the way of predictable handling or usable traction. To add to the difficulty, this section of the trail is largely exposed, making for a hot and sweaty experience. This is the hardest part of the entire ride, so if you can find some way of enjoying it, the rest of the ride will be a dream.

At mile 1.7 you enter back into the woods and the dirt returns to the singletrack, smoothing out the ride a little. Ride through a few more of those Annadel switchbacks, one of the more difficult of which features a small stand of redwood trees, standing there like an inanimate audience. Does a tree laugh in the woods when you fall off your bike?

Turn right at the next fork, where Two Quarry turns into a fire road. There's another trail sign with map here, if you need to catch your bearing. The trail cuts along a steep hillside, with the ridge above you on your right. As you climb the next 0.75 miles, the ridge slowly levels out like a giant scale beneath you. Go through a brief clearing, reenter the woods, and then come to the next fork.

There is an honest-to-goodness outhouse here and a picnic bench looking out on an expansive grassy meadow to the southeast. Beyond the meadow, the tree line reveals the results of the push to eradicate nonnative pine species from the park. The skeletons of tall pines obscure the skyline above the live green oaks.

From the picnic bench, make a left onto Marsh Trail, a fire road that climbs up and over a slight rise. On the other side of that rise appears the resplendent Ledson Marsh. The color contrasts in the marsh are a magical sight. There are many shades of green from the reeds to the grass and the fronds, and in the summer there is even red plankton that breeds on the surface of the pond.

At the next fork, head right, staying on Marsh Trail. There are a number of benches at various points around the marsh if you care to stop and enjoy the dragonflies, frogs, and other marsh-centric life.

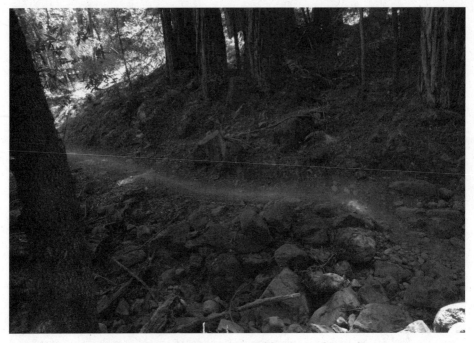

One of many technical switchbacks in the park

At the far end of the marsh you'll cross a puncheon. Shortly after that, Pig Flat Trail intersects from the left and you can extend the ride by another 1.3 miles by turning left onto Pig Flat and making the next right onto Ridge Trail. For the purpose of this ride, however, keep on Marsh Trail as it pitches upward, gets a little rough, and then picks up Ridge Trail just 0.2 miles farther.

Ridge Trail is a singletrack that makes a sharp right off Marsh Trail. It is marked with a signpost. At the turn you get the first up-close look at one of the dead pines. Notice that there is a cut running through the bark all the way around the tree. It's sad, but this is all it takes to end the life of a giant tree. Ultimately, though, this service will go a long way toward restoring the ecology of the park.

Ridge Trail is an incredible trail that was added to the park just within the last seven years. Twelve years ago, Annadel was a great park with a mediocre legal trail system and a significant network of illegal trails. Some of the illegal trails were well constructed and thought out, some were downright harmful to the park. Park officials, tired of the endless battle to close the illegal trails, instead decided to work with trail-building professionals to rework the existing trail system so that it better replicated what many park users were seeking. Many trails, like Two Quarry, were turned from wide, rough, and boringly straight affairs into twisting singletracks. Ridge Trail is a completely new addition, replacing one of the more-famous illegal trails, Upper Steve's. And it is a fantastic replacement.

This trail is 3.3 miles of singletrack perfection, turning and meandering and going on forever. It's rough and technical here, smooth and fast there, shady and exposed. Initially

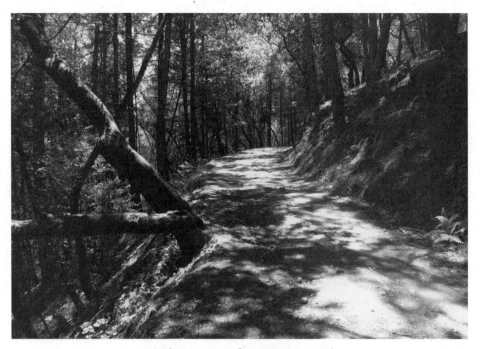

A calm portion of Two Quarry Trail

riding up onto the ridge with views of the marsh, the trail then disappears into the oaks and winds this way and that over outcroppings of volcanic rock. There are lots of ups and downs but no extended climbing, so you can really get into a groove and ride forever without tiring.

All of sudden, about two-thirds of the way into Ridge Trail, there's a picnic table, and this spot is a hot property—you'll often find it occupied by someone willing to travel this distance for some solitude.

Just after the picnic table, there's a fun downhill and another Annadel switchback, this one featuring a tiny singletrack peeling off to the left. Avoid it, staying on Ridge Trail, which enters into a dense mixed forest. Then, at the 6-mile mark, you enter in the redwood forest—a truly idyllic place, with trees towering overhead and rocks, trees, and ferns artistically scattering the floor. There are some rocks and exposed roots on the trail here, but nothing terribly technical other than a very tight switchback that might require a quick nose-wheelie/tail throw to get around.

Go by an arching fallen log, and suddenly a trail appears on the left, parallel with Ridge Trail, until they collide in a fork. This is Marsh Trail. Again, make right. Climb up a similar singletrack through a shady forest until the trees open up magnificently onto Buick Meadow. There is a bench here overlooking the meadow, and it's a great place to sit on an early morning as the peat fog slowly burns off the meadow, revealing grazing deer.

Go left at the fork onto South Burma Trail. It begins with a rocky climb up through manzanita bushes that puts you up on top of the hill. This spot is effectively 25 feet lower than the highest point in the park but serves as the top of the park because it is exposed to the sun. The trail is covered in a very light grey dust that shines like bright silver in the sun. It smells strongly of sage here, though none is visible from the trail, possibly because the visible one has been picked.

Then the descent begins. South Burma is a carryover from the old Annadel and has always been exactly the same, with only minor changes made to it throughout its life. At the top there are rollers that you can pump through, catching air off larger rock outcroppings. The trail gets rougher, the rocks smaller and more frequent the lower you descend, and the last 200 yards are possibly the roughest in the whole park.

Left at this fork will take you to Lake Ilsanjo, if you care for a 1-mile round-trip excursion to the lake. However, for this ride you will go right onto the Warren Richardson fire road, which climbs up over a slight rise and begins descending. At the next fork go right. There's a bench with good views of Lake Ilsanjo. You'll be tempted to go fast down Warren Richardson, but remember that there is a lot of traffic on this trail, including equestrian, so you must keep your speed under control. One particularly steep and rough section occurs just before the switchback where Two Quarry splits off. Some large trees that line this section feature scars from collisions. From the Two Quarry junction it's all backtracking to the car.

After the Ride

Exit Channel Drive, back onto Montgomery Road, and take a right. Drive until you come to Los Alamos Road, which Ts into Montgomery Road. There is no stop sign on Montgomery Road, so keep watch for the turn and be careful of oncoming traffic. Head 150 feet up Los Alamos and make a left onto CA 12 at the light. Drive west on CA 12 to Calistoga Road, where you'll make a right and turn into the Safeway shopping center. Tucked away in that shopping center is Su Casa Mexican Restaurant. This is an excellent economical Mexican restaurant, and it's the house sauces that really set this place apart from the rest (phone (707) 538-7937).

25

KEY AT-A-GLANCE INFORMATION

Length: 3.88 miles

Configuration: Clockwise loop

Difficulty: 5/10. Although short, this ride receives a strong rating for its technical nature.

Scenery: A lookout's view of Windsor in addition to spectacular examples of six different ecosystems

Exposure: Medium-rare. Plenty of large trees cover the majority of the ride.

Ride traffic: Park receives heavy equestrian usage. Weekend mornings and weekday evenings can be hectic.

Riding time: 1–2 hours

Access: $5 parking fee in lot

Facilities: Nice restrooms and water fountains in parking lot

GPS TRAILHEAD COORDINATES (WGS 84)

UTM Zone   10S
Easting   0520810
Northing   4263980
Latitude   N 38° 31' 33.1"
Longitude   W 122° 45' 40.7"

SHILOH RANCH REGIONAL PARK: CREEKSIDE TRAIL AND BIG LEAF LOOP

In Brief

A surprising gem in a far North Bay urburb (urban suburb), Shiloh park features not only excellent, twisty, and technical singletrack, but more large trees than you'd think could fit in such a small park.

Contact

Shiloh Ranch Regional Park
5750 Faught Road
Windsor, CA
(707) 433-1625 or 565-2041
www.sonoma-county.org/parks/pk_shilo.htm

Description

Creekside Trail trailhead is the left option of the first trail junction located at the north end of the parking lot, past the restrooms and the live oak–shaded picnic area. At time of writing, a gully washed out in the rainstorms of 2005 had yet to be repaired and a chain-link fence was diverting the trail in a very sharp and technical fashion through the bed of this creek (dry in summer). Included in this technical opener are three wooden steps, which are the most troubling piece of that puzzle.

Creekside Trail starts out as a doubletrack running alongside an old wooden post and barbed-wire fence, shaded by oaks. After about 160 yards the doubletrack turns right and starts to climb, with the creek, below to the left, as a guide. It climbs for 0.13 miles before coming

DIRECTIONS

From the Golden Gate Bridge, drive 55 miles north on US 101 to Shiloh Road. Exit right onto Shiloh Road. Drive 1.4 miles east on Shiloh Road. Turn right onto Faught Road and follow the signs to Shiloh Ranch Regional Park.

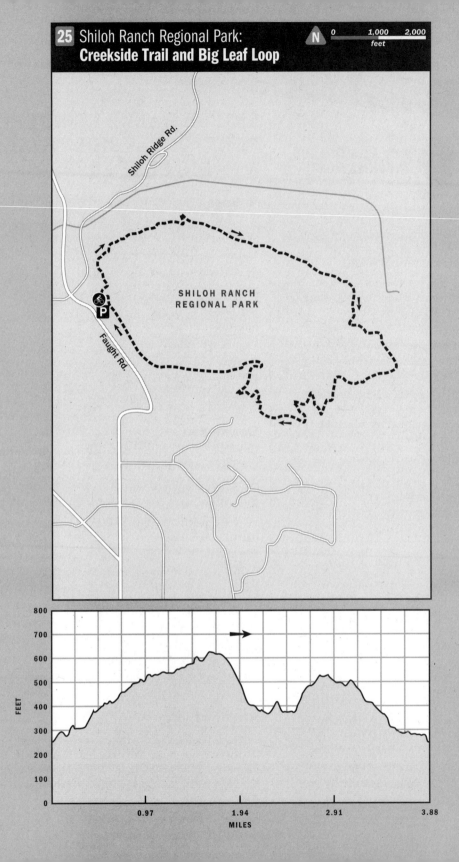

N

0   1,000   2,000
feet

SHILOH RANCH
REGIONAL PARK

Shiloh Ridge Rd.

Faught Rd.

P

800

700

600

500

400

300

200

100

0

FEET

0.97   1.94   2.91   3.88

MILES

to the next fork, marked with a signpost. Make a left onto Creekside Trail, which turns into a nice little singletrack and drops about 15 feet through madrona trees, manzanita bushes, maples, and buckeye trees, before resuming the steady climb up the hill.

This excellently maintained singletrack runs along the creek, making slight turns as the hillside and encroaching trees dictate. Human influence on the trail can be seen in the form of netting placed along exposed parts of the hillside to help prevent erosion and also in the new 20-foot-long polyurethane bridge that takes the trail across a particularly deep gulch that comes down to meet the creek.

Just after the bridge, the trail kicks up sharply for an awesome technical section, twisting through some young valley oaks. Stair steps are cut into the dirt. These make it a little more technical, but since they are dirt rather than wood, rock, or cement, they are effectively worn smooth. Traction is difficult with a thick dust layer and exposed rocks and roots.

Cresting that small climb, you enter into a bright buckeye grove, where the summer sun lights up the light green/yellow leaves and white flowers. As you progress the buckeye grove morphs into a maple grove and the green hue darkens appropriately. Within this maple grove is a technical roots section, and the best line is to the left, hugging the trunk of a live oak that meets the downhill (left) side of the trail at a 45-degree angle. Shortly after that a technical rocky section confronts you. Here, the trail narrows a lot and slips to the left of an oak that leans over the trail. You have to drop your right shoulder to clear that oak, meanwhile keeping an eye on the rock-trickery happening beneath your wheels.

The trail levels and smooths a bit after that, begging your legs for more speed. If you're not going too fast to notice, there's an old stump on the right-hand side of the trail that someone long ago carved into a single seat. It's perhaps an inauspicious section of the forest for a sightseeing seat, but it's probably a great spot to just sit and immerse oneself in the intimate sounds of the woods. And I suppose, if we're talking about seats made from still-rooted tree trunks, you gotta take them where they lie.

At about the 1-mile mark, the trees open up to grassland and coyote brush. Hard to believe, but the trail becomes even narrower and weaves a tight path through the bushes, like some natural version of the cone course at your favorite local auto-racing school.

When you reach the pond, you have the option of going around it to the right or to the left. Going right is more direct, as going left will extend your ride by just a fraction of a mile, taking the long way around this small pond. However, in the future the possibility for extension will be much larger, as park officials have begun work on a new loop, which will split off the north side of the pond and provide access to the north end of the park. The pond itself is very small, barely the size of a youth soccer field—but for a man-made reservoir, it packs a bunch of natural charm. It's teeming with life, from the reeds and the lavender flowers to the croaking frogs and dragonflies. And you'll often catch deer watering at the pond. Occasionally it gets cold enough in the winter to freeze.

Both the left-hand and right-hand routes around the pond T into Mark West Creek Trail, separately, about 20 feet from each other. Make a left onto Mark West Creek Trail. Though you'll only ride it for about 20 yards to the next fork, Mark West Creek Trail is a doubletrack that snakes away from the rest of the park to the east, where it sidles up along

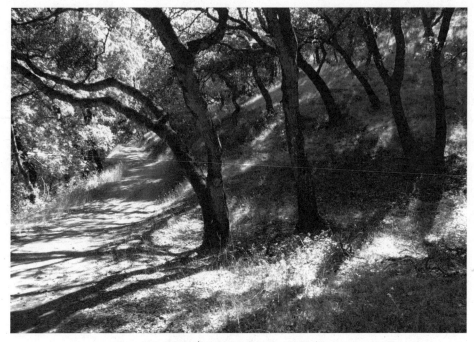

Creekside Trail starts up the hill.

Mark West Creek. This is a great out-and-back option for those looking to extend their ride by a little under 2 miles. This trail, too, will be gaining some length with the new work going on in the park, so those 2 miles could potentially be more.

At the next fork, make a right onto Ridge Trail, which is more doubletrack. From this intersection you have views down to the northern Santa Rosa/southern Windsor corridor, although the view is a bit obstructed by the trees. Ride Ridge Trail just another 0.13 miles as it snakes left around a small grove of oak trees. On the other side of those trees, you'll make a right onto Canyon Trail.

Canyon Trail is a stupendous, ultranarrow singletrack. Beware of the large poison oak bush that sits on the edge of the trail just a couple of yards from the turnoff. In fact, there is a ton of poison oak all along this trail, and in late summer the red leaves hanging from where the plants have climbed up into the oak trees form a mosaic with the greens and browns and blues in the canopy.

Initially the trail winds through the oaks on a slight downhill before it turns steep for a 42-yard section that shoots straight down the hill. Look before descending this section and stop if there is oncoming traffic, because there really is nowhere to go should you meet someone on the trail. The grade slackens a bit at the bottom before the trail runs you through a veritable ringer of oak trees, twisting every which way. The trail surface through here is very good, but there are some exposed roots that can be hard to see.

The *coup de grâce* of the whole ride comes at mile 1.7, a section of trail I like to call the Falling V. This is where the trail careens 20 feet down into a creek bed and immediately

17 feet back up the other side. The approach is all kinds of off-camber, rocky, and just plain ugly, and the bed itself is so narrow that as soon as your back wheel reaches it, the front is already on its way up the other side. This section of trail obviously got lost on its way to the Rubicon. You can definitely clear this section, if your definition of "clear" involves a 20-foot fall, a broken collar bone, and walking the rest of the way out of the park with a tacoed wheel. If you try to clear this, you'd better know how to fall.

Once through that debacle of a creek bed, you're confronted with a fork. Go left, as the right option is just a steep shortcut over top of the ridge—not legal and too steep to ride. Going left climbs you back up onto the ridge at which point the trail turns right and cuts along the ridgetop for about 30 yards before dropping down the other side. Make a left at the next fork, which is the culmination of that earlier shortcut.

For some reason the ensuing section of trail shows the strain of equestrian usage while the rest of the park doesn't (well, except for the "pies", which are everywhere): it's chewed up. The trail passes over a couple of streambeds, the first of which has a culvert, the second of which doesn't. The latter is technical but nowhere near as hard as the Falling V. There are a couple 8-by-8-inch boards thrown in, presumably to aid in crossing, but it's doubtful how much help they actually provide.

The trail climbs into an exposed section where you can catch views of the nice homes that dot the hillside to the south. At this point the trail is still singletrack, but it was obviously an old fire or logging road at some point, as you can tell by the massive cut into the hillside. The final bit up the ridge is a steep, exposed climb with the added trouble of water-diverting boards laid across the trail, but rewards come at the top.

When you reenter the trees, there is a fork; veer left and come to a bluff (don't ride too fast, eh). This is a great lookout spot with views to the west, but there is a bit of trash here from occasional kids that make the trek up at night to party. Get back on the trail, descend down from the peak, and make a left at the next fork onto South Ridge Trail doubletrack. Descend another 0.1 mile and make a right onto Big Leaf Trail. This trail makes a swooping right around a hitching post, a massive live oak, and a bench that seems to offer views of the base of the electric tower off to the left. Big Leaf Trail is a fire road that meanders down through a forest of various types of very large trees, including one humongous maple tree that may or may not have provided the leaf that is this trail's namesake. At the bottom of the hill, the trees open up and you are greeted with an expanse of vineyards and freeway noises. Make a right at the next fork and cut along the base of the hill for another 110 yards before taking the next left back into the parking lot.

After the Ride

Head south back down US 101 and exit onto Cleveland Avenue. Drive a half mile and make a right onto Piner Road; you'll find Taqueria El Sombrero Numero Dos at 810 Piner Road #A. At this spot you can replace that aching void in your stomach with a large plate of enchiladas (phone (707) 573-8278).

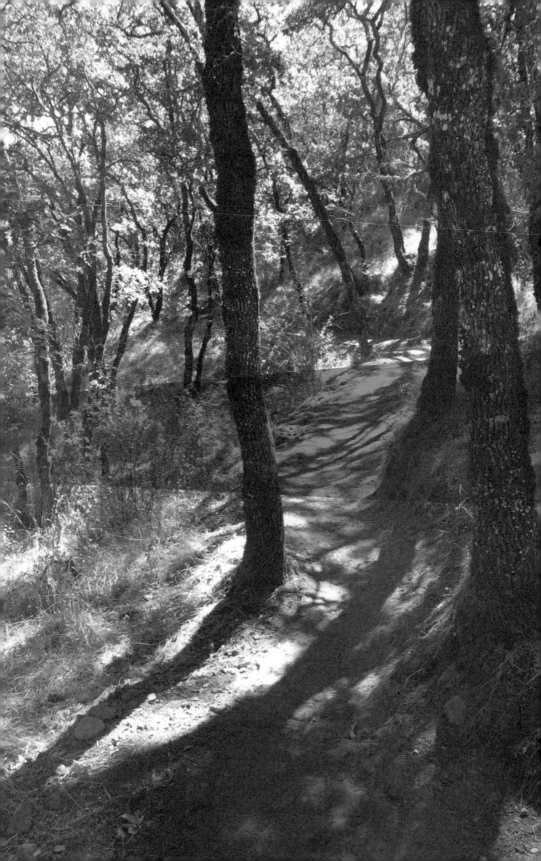

SAN FRANCISCO

26

KEY AT-A-GLANCE INFORMATION

Length: 1.6 miles

Configuration: Small out-and-back with even smaller loop at the top

Difficulty: 3/10; short and not overly technical—it's just a beautiful place to be.

Scenery: Incredible San Francisco cityscapes from the top of the city

Exposure: Minimal. Mount Davidson is covered in what some might call rain forest, but the northeastern chunk of the mountain is exposed.

Ride traffic: Absolutely minimal. Most traffic will be dog walkers and the occasional cyclocrosser doing the big city loop.

Riding time: 15–30 minutes, depending on how often you stop to take in the views

Access: Free, but located in a confusingly laid-out section of the city. Bring a street map with you.

Facilities: None.

GPS TRAILHEAD COORDINATES (WGS 84)

UTM Zone 10S
Easting 0547938
Northing 417672
Latitude N 37° 44' 18.04"
Longitude W 122° 27' 21.35"

MOUNT DAVIDSON: THE JUNGLE AT THE TOP OF SAN FRANCISCO

In Brief

The top of San Francisco. At 925 feet of elevation, Mount Davidson is the highest peak in the city and offers stunning city views in addition to some incredibly lush forest and truly enjoyable singletrack. To get to the top is something of a spiritual experience.

Description

The trailhead for this ride is midway up very steep Dalewood Way. You may have ridden to the park, in which case you will be huffing and puffing your way up Dalewood Way while also trying to scan the bushes to your left for the elusive unmarked trail and trying not to veer into the paths of the fortunately infrequent cars driving through the neighborhood. Or you may have driven,

DIRECTIONS

By car: From the Golden Gate Bridge, head south and take the CA 1/19th Avenue exit. Proceed south for 5 miles until you get to Sloat Boulevard. Turn left on Sloat Boulevard. Drive four blocks and make a left onto Portola Drive. (This is another classic San Francisco intersection, which means it is a little confusing. Make sure you don't wind up on *West Portal Drive*, which is ever so slightly to the left of Portola Drive. Go 0.8 miles up Portola Drive and make a right on Miraloma Drive. Go left on Marne Avenue, right on Juanita Way, and left on Dalewood Way. Trailhead is 250 feet up Dalewood Way on the left.

By bike: For a map of the designated bike routes that crisscross San Francisco, download the San Francisco Bike Map here: www.sfbike.org/download/map.pdf. By following this map and the city riding tips offered in the preface, you'll be able to find your way from wherever you're staying in the city to Mount Davidson. You can also use the map to connect this ride with the Mount Sutro ride (plus a couple of the other small parks contained in the city) for a serious urban mountain bike ride.

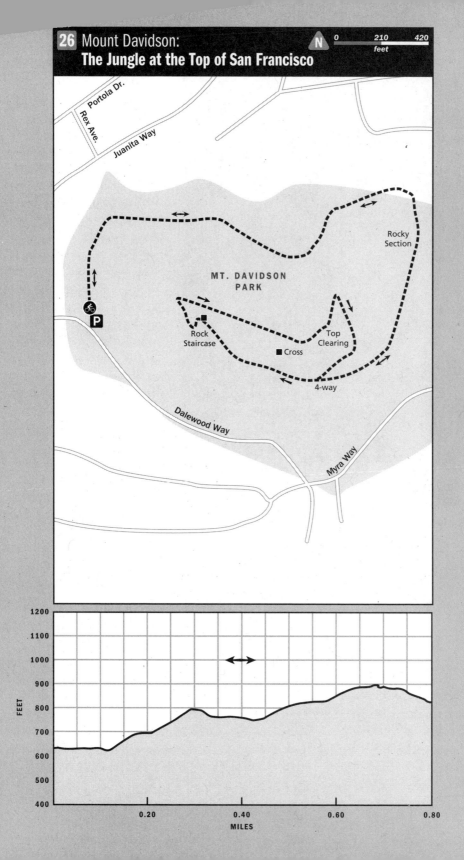

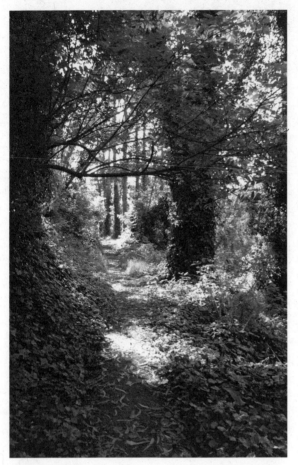

Much of Mount Davidson is covered in dense ivy.

in which case you can probably park right at the trailhead, as there is usually ample parking along Dalewood Way, except on Easter Sunday. And, when parking a car in San Francisco, always remember to curb your wheels.

The route described here essentially takes you to the top of the park in a gradually rising clockwise fashion. However, all of the trails are unmarked, so following a prescribed path can be a bit dubious. The guiding principle to this particular ride is to consistently choose the trail option in a given situation that most naturally guides you up the hillside. This means that each time you come to a fork, unless you have memorized the nameless "rights and lefts" written below, you must make a judgment call and choose the option that most gracefully progresses you up and around this tiny peak. Best rule of thumb here: avoid all sharp turns.

OK, for all you video gamers, safe crackers, professional standardized-test takers, and anyone else skilled at memorizing and employing short codes, here is a list of the directional choices you should make on this ride:

1. Trailhead off curb.
2. Right turn.
3. Right turn.
4. Right turn.
5. Left turn.
6. Stop, take in the view. North city overlook.
7. Proceed.
8. Middle option.
9. Straight at the four-way intersection.

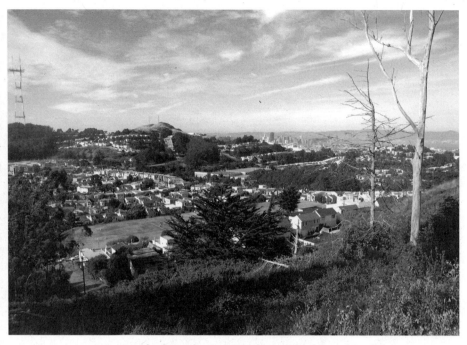

Overlooking the Twin Peaks neighborhood

10. Straight, not left.
11. Right turn at bottom of stairs.

That set of directions gets you to the top of the hill. If you were to avoid stopping to take in the view and instead wanted to proceed directly down the hill, then make a:

12. Left turn off of the plateau.
13. Sharp right.
14. Sharp left. At this point you are back on the trail you rode up on.
    Follow directions 1–8 in reverse order.

Here are some specifics to go along with that list of directions.

Directly off the curb there is a smooth log sunk into the trail at an odd angle, and if wet it will swipe your front wheel out from under you. Turns 2 through 6 take place in dense undergrowth, and blackberry bushes comprise a lot of this, so wear some sleeves and take care not to fall off. There are also some rather large tree stumps hidden within these brambles, and cutting certain turns might wind up giving you more than a few thorny scratches.

Between turns 8 and 9, there are two technical rocky sections; the first is uphill and roughly three yards long, and the second is downhill and roughly two yards long.

The stairs mentioned in number 11 are a flight of 12, constructed of rock, and pretty steep. If you're on a full-suspension bike and are a confident sort, ride down them. If not,

I'd suggest hopping off and portaging down. There's no particularly good line, and crashing usually hurts, even in beautiful places such as this.

Once you find yourself at the top of the hill, stop and have a look around. The plateau is about the size of half a football field, and it offers incredible views of the city on most sides, particularly to the eastern side, where you can soak in San Francisco's downtown skyline. This would be a great place to plan a romantic picnic or maybe an intervention. You've probably read about the 103-foot tall cross at the top of the hill. Services are held on Easter every year, and that's probably the only day you'll ever find this park crowded.

Another great tactic would be to just scrap these directions and head up to Mount Davidson and get lost, which wouldn't be such a bad thing. The park is so small that you're bound to make it to the top somehow, within an hour of trying, even if you find yourself summarily spat out into the surrounding neighborhood or pushing your way up an impossibly steep section after various wrong turns. Spending time traipsing around even a small gem of a park such as this is time well spent.

After the Ride

Head back down the hill to 19th Avenue, turn right (north), and drive 15 blocks to Judah Street. Turn right on Judah Street, drive to 9th Avenue, and turn left. On the left-hand side of 9th Avenue at Judah Street is a great restaurant/sports bar called Cybelle's Front Room. Offering beer, gourmet pizzas, and American and Italian fare, this is a great place to eat. I can recommend everything on the menu, because it is all delicious. But if pressed I'd say go with the club sandwich. It's mighty good (phone (415) 665-8088).

27

KEY AT-A-GLANCE INFORMATION

Length: 3.56 miles

Configuration: Out-and-back

Difficulty: 7/10; some technical switchbacks; climb/descend 'em if you can

Scenery: Glimpsed through the trees: northwest San Francisco

Exposure: Rare. *If* it's sunny in San Francisco when you go up, you won't feel it through the dense tree cover.

Ride traffic: Medium-high in the evenings, otherwise light

Riding time: 0.75–1.25 hours

Access: Parking in San Francisco is always tight, but the city is also small enough that you can just ride to the park anyway.

Facilities: None

GPS TRAILHEAD COORDINATES (WGS 84)

UTM Zone 10S
Easting 0548066
Northing 4179535
Latitude N 37° 45' 40.98"
Longitude W 122° 27' 17.85"

MOUNT SUTRO: MOUNT SUTRO OUT-AND-BACK

In Brief

Resurrected in 2005 thanks to the Mount Sutro Trail Stewards, it is believed that this trail system dates back to before 1900, and it is suspected that they are part of an old system of logging trails. They were discovered during a survey of the open space above the UCSF medical center. San Francisco routinely ranks in the top five in terms of population density, and it's hard to believe that a place as beautiful as Mount Sutro can exist—and such a quiet existence at that! You won't regret visiting this little nugget of wild terrain. Ride it out and back, or connect it with the Mount Davidson ride, as described on pages 144–148.

Contact

www.natureinthecity.org/mtsutro.php

Description

Farnsworth Lane is a tiny little dead-end street tucked up behind the UCSF medical center. The trailhead for this ride is located at the gravelly terminus of Farnsworth Lane and, with its drooping chain gate in among dense and drooping branches, could be mistaken for the eerie

DIRECTIONS

Mount Sutro is located behind the Parnassus Campus of the University of California San Francisco (USFC) Medical Center on Parnassus Avenue in the Inner Sunset neighborhood of San Francisco. From UCSF, head east on Parnassus Avenue three long blocks until you make a right onto Woodland Avenue. Follow Woodland Avenue as it makes a right-hand U-turn through the neighborhood and then make a left onto Belmont Avenue, which hits Woodland Avenue at a diagonal. From Belmont Avenue, turn right onto Edgewood Avenue and follow that as it turns into Farnsworth Lane, which almost instantly dead-ends at the trailhead.

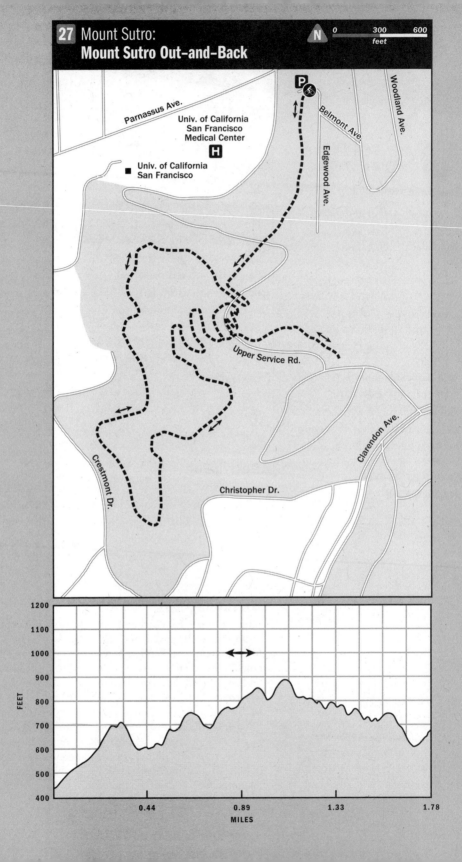

driveway of some much more remote private estate. Step over the gate and through the branches, though, and you find yourself on a nice little shaded singletrack with the medical buildings visible through the trees.

From the gate, head left up the hill. The trail forks a couple of times in the first 100 yards, but follow the trail closest to the private fence on your left, and the trail ramps steeply for 20 feet and dumps you in a long, narrow parking lot. This is called Surge Lot, and no you can't park here for your ride because it is UCSF permit only. Ride up through the lot and make a left onto Medical Center Way. Ride about 0.15 miles and make your next paved right turn onto a service road that heads up to some water tanks that are the size of buildings.

Don't get carried away and ride up to the tanks, because the trail actually picks up again right inside the apex of this turn. This unmarked trail is called Historic Trail, and within the ensuing short but epic mile and a half it will definitely be written into the history of your life.

From the pavement, the trail drops a few yards before leveling out on the ridge above Medical Center Way, which will gradually disappear from view within the next couple hundred feet as the trail winds around the northwest side of the peak of the mountain. Immediately after leaving the pavement, you spin happily through amazing lush ferns, vines, and eucalyptus trees, with the medical center just barely visible through the trees.

Make a left at the next fork and commence the climbing! You won't be tired this early in the ride, but the option to the right is a small clearing from which you can enjoy some of the views of San Francisco's Sunset district through the dense eucalyptus trees. The other greenbelt seen across the way is good old GGP (Golden Gate Park), a nice place to visit, but you wouldn't want to mountain bike there.

Yes, there are some intense views to be had here, but this is less about the view and more about the trail itself, because it is awesome. The Mount Sutro Trail Stewards and associated volunteers have done an outstanding job in prepping this trail. The surface is nice and smooth with only a few very small stumps and minor root systems to add some flavor. There are a couple large rock outcroppings impinging on the trail, and it's fun to arch your body around them, keeping your soft bits away from the jagged edges. The trail isn't all that technical at this point, but there is one very good reason to keep your concentration on it: two parallel pipes running diagonally and downhill across the trail about a foot above it. Hitting these things wrong will send you careening down the hillside; at least that's what happened the one time I tried to jump over them. I don't recommend you try either, unless you're of Hans Rey's ilk.

Make a right at the next fork, and in another hundred feet come to a four-way intersection, where you'll turn left. This is the top of the ridge. The peak is still above you to the east, and you're surrounded by trees, but otherwise you'd have 280-degree views. The next fork comes very quickly; make a right. Then suddenly another paved road appears out of nowhere, and the trail Ts into it. This is Nike Road. Turn left and ride up, going past a placard designating the area a San Francisco Rotary summit garden (the Rotary Club donated a very generous sum for the purpose of eradicating invasive plant species grown rampant in the open space and replanting the area with native species). Hop off your bike and

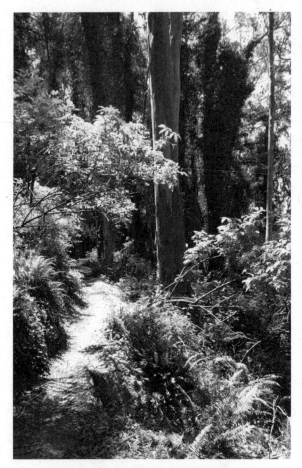

Singletrack cutting through lush forest, right in the middle of the city

jump over the chain gate running across Nike Road, which turns to gravel about 15 yards later.

The gravel is deep, loose pea gravel, and it can wash out your front wheel just slightly less efficiently than sand if you're not careful. At mile 1.1 turn right at the next fork and you come into to a wide-open area framed by eucalyptus at the top of the mountain and the extended portion of the summit garden. You may want to have your picnic here.

Past the gardens at the north end of the clearing, the trail continues to the left of some large boulders. This is North Ridge Trail, and this is where it gets technical, with an awesome switchback-strewn singletrack downhill. Go straight at the four-way intersection and right at the following fork. This is a very tight section through some trees, and it's a cool little chicane.

You'll come to a paved road at the bottom of these switchbacks, and it is Medical Center Way (the same road you were on earlier). Be careful and cross directly to the other side, where Fairy Gates Trail continues between two large eucalyptus trees. It's a tight reentry, and the trail drops steeply right away through some lush greenery, including blackberry bushes (though work is underway to reduce the impact of blackberry bushes in the open space, so these may have been removed when you make it up here).

If you're still in control, make a left at the fork. This is a small extra loop, and it is totally worth it, because you're going to descend down through some of the tightest switchbacks ever! You weave through the dense foliage and small trees. This is such a fun section for being only 0.13 miles long. It loops back around to Medical Center Way, and when you hit the road, turn left onto the dirt path running alongside, ride back up to the trail, and make that left back onto the trail—only this time make a right at the first fork, instead of a left.

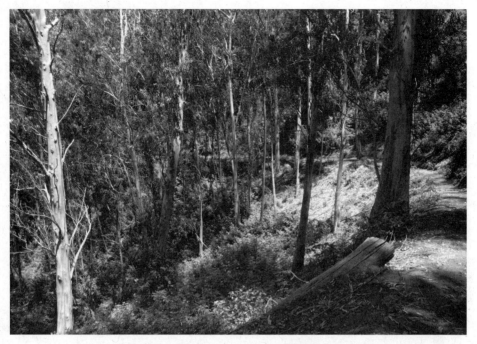

Despite its location, it's not uncommon to find the park as quiet as this.

The trail levels out a bit and runs along the hillside. There are three 8 to 15 feet rocky sections that are difficult, if not impossible, to ride. If you don't want to dismount to cross these, you'll have to do some hopping. The trail ends at the mouth of a private driveway off Johnstone Road.

If you are interested, you can ride a little farther on the pavement to the base of the big red-and-white Sutro Tower. Just make a left onto Johnstone Road, ride down, and make a right onto Clarendon Road. Ride up Clarendon Road to the next left and carefully cross into the neighborhood on the other side. Look up; that's Sutro Tower.

Now, turn around and ride all that good stuff back to Farnsworth Lane. Or continue on to Mount Davidson (see page 144).

After the Ride

Get back on Parnassus Avenue and head east to Cole Valley. Turn left on Cole Street. From this street you have many good options, including Kezar Bar & Restaurant at 900 Cole Street (phone (415) 681-7678), Burgermeister at 86 Carl Street (phone (415) 566-1274), or the supersecret no-name no-signs sushi restaurant located somewhere in that area. Also good are Boulange de Cole Valley (phone (415) 242-2442), Citrus Club Thai Restaurant on Haight Street (phone (415) 387-6366), or Cha Cha Cha's for tapas, also on Haight (phone (415) 386-7670).

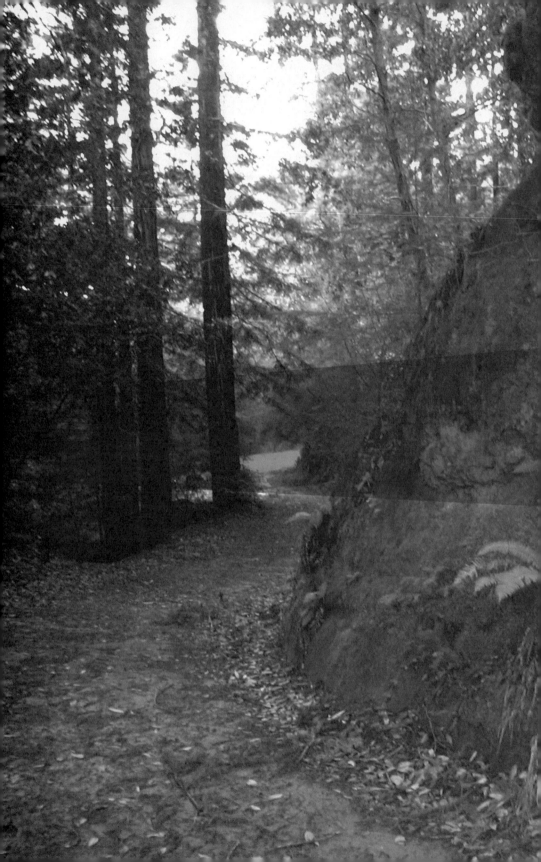

SOUTH BAY

28

PACIFICA: SWEENEY RIDGE LOOP

KEY AT-A-GLANCE INFORMATION

Length: 6.7 miles

Configuration: Out-and-back horseshoe

Difficulty: 7/10; not technical but steep

Scenery: On a clear day, views all around: east to San Francisco Bay, west to Pacifica and the ocean, north to San Bruno Mountain. Amazing western views during sunset.

Exposure: Well-done; no trees to shade or protect from wind

Ride traffic: Low

Riding time: 2–3 hours

Access: Ample free parking at Shelldance Nursery parking lot

Facilities: None at trailhead; portable restroom at Nike Missile Silo

In Brief

Rewheeling the steps of 18th-century Spanish explorer Gaspar de Portolá, this ride takes you up the steep Mori Ridge Trail, first to a very 20th-century abandoned missile site and then on to where Portolá and his men first sighted San Francisco Bay.

Description

Although this book champions the sanctity of the dirt and the directions indicate to start this ride at the trailhead in the Shelldance Nursery parking lot, you might strongly consider starting this ride in the parking lot of Pacifica State Beach (**www.parks.ca.gov/default.asp?page_id=524**) and ride the 2.5-mile paved bike path up the beach and then to the trailhead. Your legs will thank you for warming them up prior to the steep climb up Mori Ridge Trail, and you'll also get a chance to experience more of Pacifica.

The driveway leading up to the trailhead in the Shelldance Nursery parking lot is a little obscure. Whether riding or driving, look for large, colorful signs declaring ORCHIDS from CA 1. There is a miniscule sign in a field near (not even *at*, just near) the base of this driveway indicating that this is Mori Ridge Trail. You are guaranteed not to see this sign, so just follow the orchid signs instead. Once you get up to the large gravel parking lot, though, there is a large Golden Gate National Recreation Area sign in the northwest corner declaiming the area as Sweeney Ridge.

GPS TRAILHEAD COORDINATES (WGS 84)

UTM Zone 10S
Easting 0545720
Northing 4163260
Latitude N 37° 37' 1.9"
Longitude W 122° 28' 54.8"

DIRECTIONS

Take Interstate 280 south from Daly City 6.5 miles and exit CA 1 toward Pacifica. Follow CA 1 for 4 miles through the town of Pacifica. Past the Sharp Park Golf Course, make a U-turn at the Reina Del Mar Avenue and drive about 200 yards back up CA 1 until you see the signs for the Shelldance Nursery. Drive up the driveway into the Shelldance Nursery parking lot.

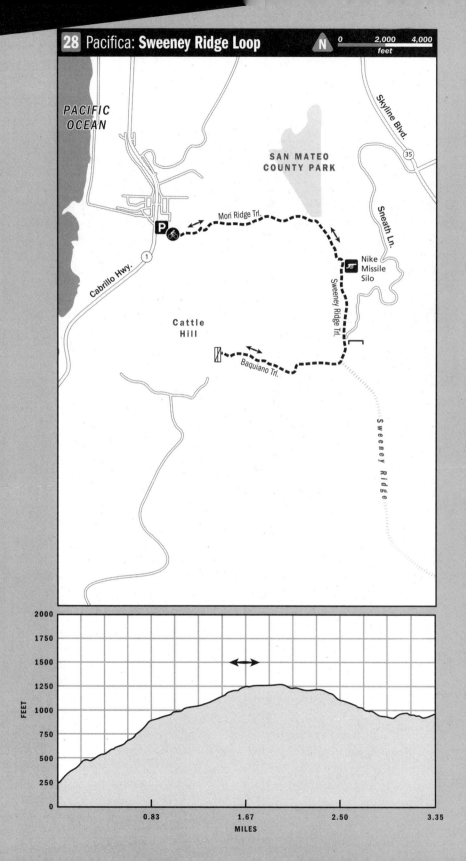

N

0   2,000   4,000
feet

PACIFIC
OCEAN

Skyline Blvd.

SAN MATEO
COUNTY PARK

35

Mori Ridge Trl.

P

Sneath Ln.

Nike
Missile
Silo

Cabrillo Hwy.

1

Sweeney Ridge Trl.

Cattle
Hill

Baquiano Trl.

Sweeney Ridge

2000
1750
1500
1250
1000
750
500
250
0

FEET

0.83   1.67   2.50   3.35
MILES

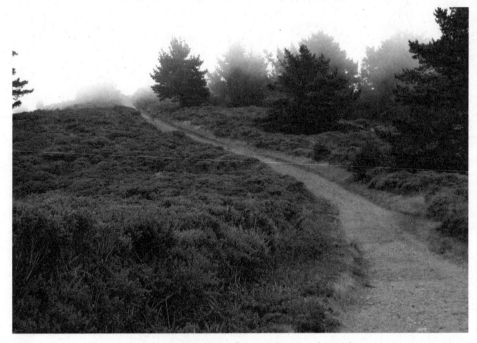

Heavy fog adds a bit of mysticism to this ridge.

Proceed up the gravel road just to the left of that sign. The gravel extends only a few yards past the sign before turning into dirt fire road. The climbing begins right away. If your legs aren't warm, you may find yourself walking this section, but don't get too frustrated, since within the first 35 yards, you come to a closed white metal gate. There is a pedestrian opening to the left of the gate, but it's too tight a squeeze for most handlebars, so you'll have to dismount and carry your bike through.

Thanks to the steep early climbing, great views come early on this ride as Pacifica quickly splays out below. Early views of the Pacifica Pier—popular for fishing—and Sharp Golf Course lie to the north, and the hilly, jagged coast lies to the south. Close at hand is some classic coastal chaparral.

Mori Ridge Trail runs up the ridgeline, trying to be as steep and straight as possible, just like any good fire-cut-turned-trail worth its salt. With proper gearing, warm legs, and a positive understanding that the steepest portion only lasts for the first 1.3 miles, you should get up this hill with a minimum of fuss. Trail surface is very good, hard-pack dirt, with very little in the way of loose rocks and sand.

Coyote brush dots the grassland, and there are a few clusters of pine trees here and there. With the exception of one large pine, most of these trees are short and squat in order to deal with the regular high winds ripping over the ridge. A wide variety of colorful wildflowers line the trail, including a significant amount of white daisies blooming throughout summer.

At mile 1.21 Sweeney Ridge Trail joins from the left. Continue right on Mori Ridge Trail. You've gained 700 feet in elevation from the parking lot at this point, and just

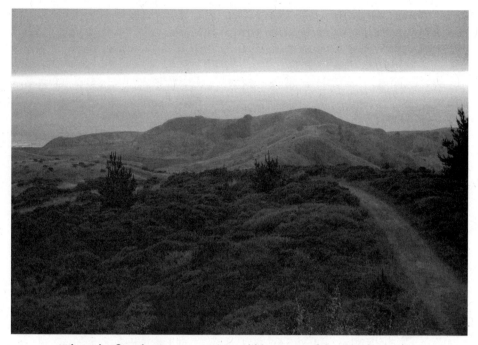

When the fog clears, you get incredible views of the Pacific Ocean.

another 250 feet will bring you to the top of the ridge. From this intersection the trail weaves left and then right, gets steep for about 15 yards, and then hits pavement. The paved road that Mori Ridge Trail Ts into is Sweeney Ridge Trail, and before you get to it, if you're not looking down because your tongue is caught in your gears, you'll see one of the buildings of the Nike Missile Site.

Checking out this abandoned military complex is a must, so detour right on Sweeney Ridge and ride over to the buildings. There are 24 of these Nike Missile Sites scattered throughout the Bay Area. They were originally designed to provide ground-to-air missile protection for the city of San Francisco and surrounding areas. They were decommissioned back in the 1970s and exist in various levels of decay. The Sweeney Ridge site, #SF-51C, is in sad shape. The cinder-brick buildings remain, but the windows have all been shattered and most of the buildings seem to have suffered fire at some point or other. All told, there are four buildings plus an old guard booth and a 30-foot-diameter cement landing pad, presumably for helicopters. The building shells, some metal ducting, and an odd piece of equipment remain. When the fog rolls in, this complex has a very eerie quality, the prevalence of graffiti lending it a Mad Max sort of feel. Just a bit of weird up in the pretty hills.

When you've gotten the Max Rockatansky out of your blood, get back onto paved Sweeney Ridge Trail and head south (had you turned directly off Mori Ridge Trail, it would have been left). After about 0.13 miles, a solid yellow line appears in the middle of the path, which looks funny since the path is one lane wide at best. It's basically to direct the cycle traffic that makes it up onto the ridge.

At the next fork go right on Sweeney Ridge Trail, which turns into dirt, while Sneath Lane is the paved path that takes a sharp left and shoots down the hill. After about 45 yards down the trail, you'll make a right. There is a bench here facing west, although the view isn't so good when the fog has rolled in.

Next you'll come to a small fork on the left with a sign pointing you to the Portolá Discovery Site. Head up to the small clearing and check out the view (if the fog permits it) east to the San Francisco Bay and San Francisco Airport, and northeast to San Bruno Mountain. At the north end of the clearing is a rock monument briefly outlining that this is where Gaspar de Portolá and his men first sighted the bay on November 4, 1769. Opposite that is another stone monument, this one dedicated to a Carl Patrick McCarthy, who worked to give the historical location its public due.

Get back on the trail, ride down to the next fork, and make a right onto Baquiano Trail. This is another fire road and will be the third leg of this horseshoe-shaped ride. Baquiano Trail begins descending right away, making a sharp right 110 yards past the fork. In all, it descends a couple hundred feet before climbing over a slight roller and then up to a gate.

The rusty old red gate is broken and sitting open. This is the official turnaround point of the ride. Just beyond the gate, the trail forks, but neither of these trails are legal for bikes. Oddly, though, as of this writing, the usage rights weren't posted anywhere on the trail, and only if one were familiar with the park map (also not available at the trailhead) would one know not to ride on these trails. It's feasible, if you didn't feel like riding back around the horseshoe, that you could walk the roughly 0.3 miles down the trail on the left, which would place you at the top of Fassler Avenue, which you could then ride down to CA 1 and wind up just a little north of your starting point at Pacifica State Beach.

But since you're a trooper, you should backtrack to the Shelldance Nursery parking lot, giving yourself another opportunity to enjoy the amazing views of Pacifica from Mori Ridge Trail. It's much easier heading back the other way, since it's practically all downhill. All told, mountain bikers would really benefit if the park were to invest in a more elaborate, maintained trail system. Having just a winding singletrack alternative to Mori Ridge Trail would knock its difficulty rating from a 7 to a 6 and make it just a little more fun.

After the Ride

Drive back north on CA 1 exit Paloma Avenue and go west back under the freeway. Turn left onto Francisco Boulevard and drive four and a half blocks to Pacifica Thai Cuisine for some spicy soup to warm you up after what was probably a fog-soaked excursion up in the Pacifica hills (phone (415) 355-1678).

29

Length: 6.66 miles

Configuration: Counterclockwise loop with 0.3-mile out-and-back

Difficulty: 8/10; technical descent plus 1,600+ feet of climbing

Scenery: Incredible redwood forest and valley vistas

Exposure: Medium-rare. This park is all about the dense, shady redwood forest, but there are some exposed sections here and there, particularly on the climb back up Harkins Ridge Trail.

Ride traffic: Medium. Somewhat remote location ensures mostly outdoors-savvy crowds.

Riding time: 1.75–2.5 hours

Access: Free parking for up to 40 cars

Facilities: Restrooms and ranger station are located at parking lot in case of emergencies.

GPS TRAILHEAD COORDINATES (WGS 84)

UTM Zone   10S
Easting   0558583
Northing   4144805
Latitude   N 37° 27' 0.4"
Longitude   W 122° 20' 15.2"

PURISIMA CREEK REDWOODS: WHITTEMORE WONDERLAND

In Brief

Whittemore Gulch Trail is a seasonal trail and is subject to long closures (to mountain bikes and equestrians) throughout the wet season, but when it *is* open, it truly is a wonderland. Possibly some of the best singletrack switchbacks to be had in the whole North Bay, Whittemore Gulch Trail is a fantastic slalom ride down the face of a plush hillside. There are incredible long-range views in this park, but it's all about being up close and personal with various colors of the thriving vegetation that surrounds you on all sides.

Contact

Purisima Creek Redwoods Open Space Preserve
Midpeninsula Regional Open Space District
330 Distel Circle
Los Altos, CA 94022-1404
(650) 691-1200
www.openspace.org/preserves/pr_purisima.asp

Description

Do a quick lap around North Ridge parking lot (taking care not to get run over, of course) and make sure that your equipment is in working order. This ride begins with a challenging descent down Whittemore Gulch Trail, and you don't want mechanical issues to disrupt this ride.

DIRECTIONS

From San Francisco, head approximately 13 miles south on Interstate 280 until you come to CA 92/San Mateo Road. Exit CA 92 toward Half Moon Bay. Cross over the Crystal Springs Reservoir and drive 2 miles until you come to the intersection with CA 35/Skyline Boulevard. Turn left onto Skyline Boulevard and drive 5.4 miles south until you see the sign for the Purisima Creek Redwoods Open Space Park North Ridge parking lot on the right.

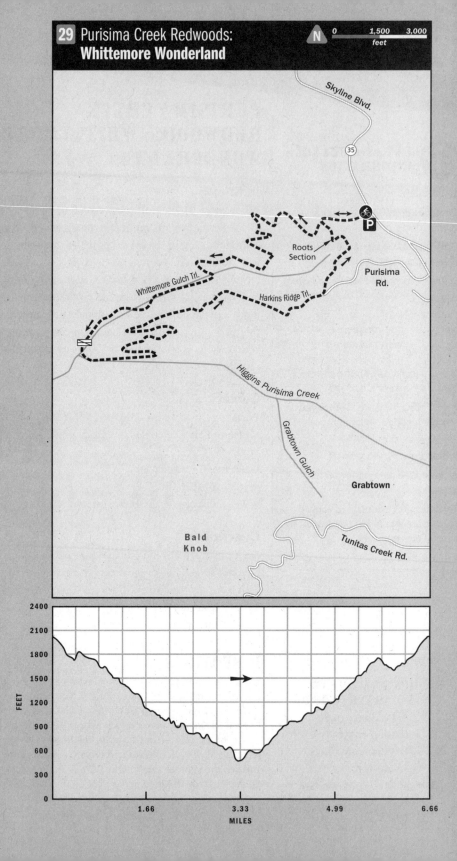

N

0   1,500   3,000
feet

Skyline Blvd.

35

Roots
Section

Whittemore Gulch Trl.

Harkins Ridge Trl.

Purisima
Rd.

Higgins Purisima Creek

Grabtown Gulch

Grabtown

Bald
Knob

Tunitas Creek Rd.

2400
2100
1800
1500
1200
900
600
300
0

FEET

1.66   3.33   4.99   6.66

MILES

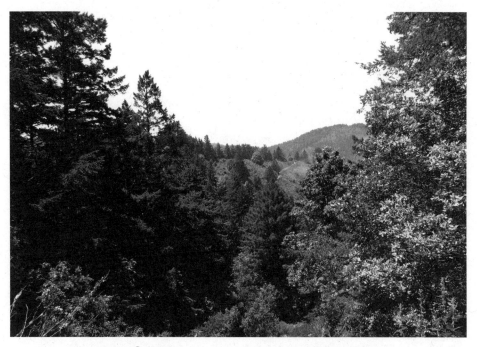

Dense forest is a common sight along Skyline Ridge.

Gate PC01 is located on the south end of the parking lot. There is a trail sign there displaying a blown-up map of the park and offering personal maps. This sign will indicate whether or not Whittemore Gulch is open on the day of your ride. There is also a Web site that tells of trail closures (**www.openspace.org/preserves/pr_purisima.asp**) that you can check before venturing to the park.

North Ridge Trail begins just to the left of the sign. Pass through the gate, and the fun begins with a great, rolling doubletrack downhill. There are some rollers off which to grab some air and test out your suspension (or lack thereof). A quarter mile into the descent, take the center option at the three-way fork, staying on North Ridge Trail.

At mile 0.7 you come to the next fork. This is Whittemore Gulch Trail, and it is protected by a small gate, which is closed when the trail is deemed unfit for riding. Please don't poach this trail when it is closed. What's good for the trail is good for the rider, and basically not only is it damaging to the trail and ecosystem to ride this trail when wet, but it's also not enjoyable in the slightest because the mud is very slick and what was a tight, difficult descent becomes impossible. Oh, and the fines are steep.

That said, this is an absolutely incredible trail, featuring countless switchbacks down through countless trees and countless types of vegetation. The trail is very skinny, thanks in large part to the fact that it's never ridden in foul weather. The vegetation plays a huge part in this as well, and left unchecked it would probably swallow the trail in the space of a season. Lush vegetation in Northern California almost always brings with it poison oak, and this park is no exception. It's really a crapshoot whether or not you'll find a great deal of the plant encroaching on the trail, as it does get cleared occasionally. There is bound to be some, and if you're allergic and don't want to have to worry about slowing to examine every bush on your descent, then take precautions: removable sleeves and pant legs are one option. Otherwise you can pretreat with one of the products on the market and also bring along some post-exposure treatment to keep in the car for after the ride.

Trail surface is smooth, with just a few exposed roots and rocks here and there, so you don't have to pin your focus to that but can instead scan ahead to the next switchback. Something to watch out for are slick spots on the trail. As the park is situated on the west side of the mountain that receives a great deal of coastal wind and fog, the moisture levels are very high, and in the shadiest places the trail surface retains moisture throughout even the warmest days. Because there isn't enough moisture to saturate much deeper than a few inches, it means that these sections are slick.

The myth goes that there is no stable number of switchbacks on Whittemore Gulch Trail, and you'll get a different count every time you ride it. Well, OK, there are somewhere between 3 and 3,000 switchbacks. Good? Basically, I could tell you the exact number, but what fun would it be to have a countdown running through your mind while you're trying to enjoy the trail? There are *many* switchbacks, and each one entices the motor skills in its own unique way.

From the usually mist-shrouded gate at the top, you drop off the ridge veering left through the trees toward the first switchback. From that point on, the trail unfolds with the beautiful irregularity of an interpretive dance performance. Speeding forward, turning, falling, jumping, weaving, turning, turning, turning. As you descend the hill the vegetation is constantly changing around you, from virtually rain forest to dry chaparral, all within spaces of dozens of feet. Above halfway down the hill, when you hit the chaparral and your tires are rolling over arid, yellow soil, you get views up and down the hill, seeing the tree line you just emerged from and that into which you will momentarily disappear. There is one fork that pops up within the first 0.6 miles; make a left to stay on Whittemore Gulch Trail. Near the bottom of the trail on the run back into the woods, you will ride through sheets of bright white poison hemlock hanging over the trail.

Once you reenter the woods, you hit a puncheon at mile 2.3. It officially signals the end of the twisties; you've just dropped about 1,000 feet in elevation in just over a mile of switchbacks. Cross the trail's namesake creek over the slick, wet puncheon and then begin a fun, relatively straight descent. It's a fairly steep descent through the redwood forest, with the creek on the right and a fern-covered hillside on the left. The beauty of this area relates to the complex contours of the terrain, highlighted by the many different layers of canopy. When the sun is shining, the ravine is filled with a dark green glow as the rays bounce around throughout the canopy.

There are a couple of rollers, including one uphill spike that drops off sharply on the other side, revealing a rare rocky section. The blind crest and suddenly choppy surface are a dangerous combination, so exercise caution on these rollers.

Sadly, the descent has to end, and once you reach the gate at the bottom of the hill, you know that time has come. The gate opens up to a clearing, and passing through the gate is like stepping out of a building. Ride through this small meadow and enter back into the woods and immediately come to a fork. Take a left onto Harkins Ridge Trail heading back toward the North Ridge parking lot, listed on the sign as being some 3.3 miles distant. The right turn leads down to a bridge, which in turn leads to park gate PC05 and the Purisima Creek Road parking lot. This is the most popular access point to the park, and it is usually quite congested. There are restrooms in Purisima Creek parking lot.

Harkins Ridge Trail is a rigorous climb back up the hill. It's a doubletrack trail that is much more exposed than Whittemore Gulch and is situated on the south ridge above the gulch, affording some incredible views of the redwood and Douglas fir forest unrolling to the south. At mile 4.35 the trail makes a wide right-hand switchback, cutting around a cluster of yellow-orange California false lupine. This is probably the most scenic view of the entire ride.

Stay left on Harkins Ridge Trail at the next two forks. The bulk of the climbing is over by the second of these forks, and the trail levels out, but it gets a little rockier to keep it interesting. Then at mile 6.25, after you reenter the woods, there is a ten-yard-long technical section of wet, exposed roots. There is a stream running through here that keeps the trail constantly muddy, and with the shade working to obscure your vision (especially if you've got sunglasses on) then it's ten-to-one odds you have to dismount and walk.

Make a right at the next fork, and you're back on North Ridge Trail and it's a 0.3-mile climb back up to the parking lot.

After the Ride

Although a little pricey and only open from Wednesday to Sunday, The Mountain House Restaurant at 13808 Skyline Boulevard (phone (650) 851-8541) is an attraction in its own right. Go to the bar when it opens at 5 p.m. and order some appetizers and a glass of wine. Or bring some nice clothes and moist wipes to clean up after the ride, do it right, and get a reservation for dinner. It's just a little over a mile down Skyline Boulevard from the trail-head; how can you refuse?

PURISIMA CREEK REDWOODS: GRABTOWN GULCH LOOP

In Brief

If you're interested in learning to speak redwood, then this is the full-immersion program. Grabtown Gulch is sunk deep in a 50-to-60-year-old redwood forest, and this loop treats you with a fast singletrack descent down through the trees to Purisima Creek and then a climb back up a twisty doubletrack that's not too steep to allow you to enjoy sights, sounds, and smells of the forest that surrounds you.

Contact

Purisima Creek Redwoods Open Space Preserve
Midpeninsula Regional Open Space District
330 Distel Circle
Los Altos, CA 94022-1404
(650) 691-1200
www.openspace.org/preserves/pr_purisima.asp

Description

Gate PC04—your trailhead—appears suddenly out of the dense redwood forest as you drive west down Tunitas Creek Road from Skyline Boulevard. It is illuminated by the sun in an unusual clearing of the trees, sitting

DIRECTIONS

From San Francisco, head approximately 13 miles South on Interstate 280 until you come to CA 92/San Mateo Road. Exit CA 92 toward Half Moon Bay. Cross over the Crystal Springs Reservoir and drive 2 miles until you come to the intersection with CA 35/Skyline Boulevard. Turn left onto Skyline Boulevard and drive 6 miles south to the intersection of CA 35 and Tunitas Creek Road. Turn right onto Tunitas Creek Road, which is a narrow, twisting, undivided road set deep in the woods. Drive approximately 1.8 miles west on Tunitas Creek Road to gate PC04, which will be on the right. There is no parking lot, but plenty of pulloffs are along the side of the road.

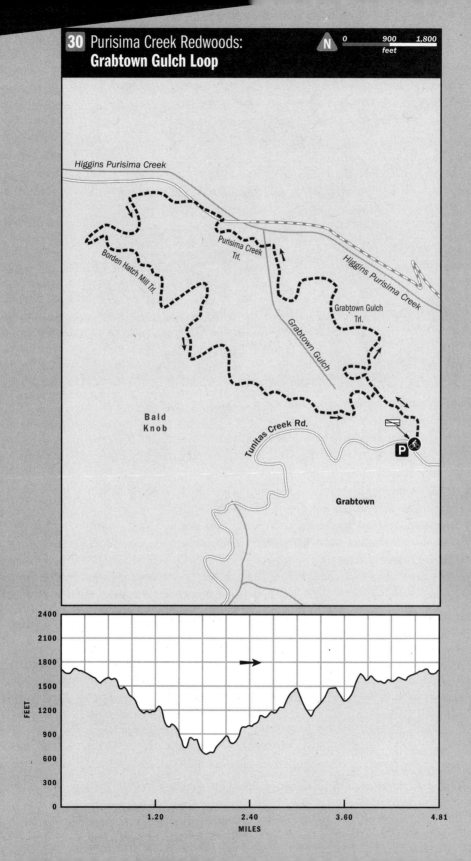

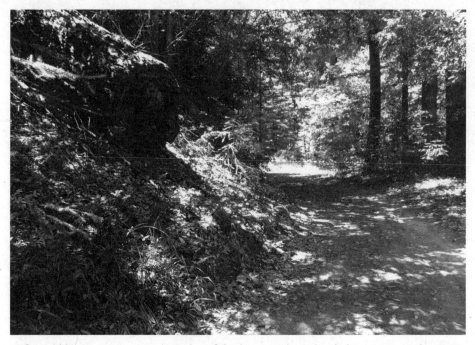

A few old logs remain as a reminder of the logging these lands have seen in the past.

opposite a private driveway and not nearly as cluttered with visitors' cars since most park users aggregate at the Higgins–Purisima Road parking lot or one of the two Skyline Boulevard parking lots.

Enter through the gate and give your bike a check, since you'll be heading downhill right off the bat and you won't want to miss any of the flow by having to stop and adjust something. You will, however, *want* to miss a run-in with a large redwood tree, and since Grabtown Gulch flirts with a lot of them, you'd better make sure your skewers are tight and your brakes working.

It begins as a slight downhill, rolling ever deeper into the woods. You pass an empty clearing on the left that is apparently a tract expecting a home and is well marked as private. The speed picks up, and the trail offers up a few slight rollers to get a little air off of.

After 0.3 miles, you come to another small clearing and a fork. Go right onto Grabtown Gulch, and immediately you are immersed in the forest and heading down a steep, somewhat wide singletrack. The trail makes a sharp left, a smooth swooping right-hander that's sticky enough to allow you to pull some serious Gs, and then another sharp left. All around you are ferns and other sorts of lush forest-floor flora. There is some poison oak, but it's not grabbing out at you.

The trail descends steeply, following the contours of the hill. It winds just enough to make it fun. Aside from a couple of small streams that run across the trail in deep, muddy gouges, the trail surface itself is quite smooth. Keep your eyes open as the changing light conditions under the canopy can hide those gouges, which are deep enough to grab a 26-inch wheel. A quick wheelie will get you through no problem. As with the rest of the park, there are small sections of trail that retain moisture throughout even the hottest days and remain slick, so watch out for these as well. Semislick cross-country racing tires aren't recommended in this park because of these slick spots. A good knobby will help prevent your bike from spitting out from under you at an inopportune moment (not that there is ever an opportune moment for that). There are also a few false turns—cuts made by a tractor—that jut off the trail at odd angles. Although these cuts are usually full of forest debris and don't resemble the actual trail, it's worth a warning to avoid getting all wrapped up in the descent and mistaking one of these cuts for the trail itself and finding yourself careening head-first down a ravine.

One particularly steep section dives into a really sharp left-hander, and it's easy to get too much speed and risk blowing

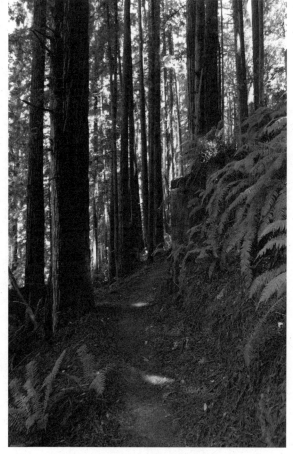

Grabtown Gulch Trail, flirting with the young redwoods

out the end of this turn. And, of course, take precautions in case another park-goer is just the other side of the turn. Almost all cyclists opt to descend this trail, so you won't meet too many of them coming the other way, but hikers frequent this trail equally in both directions, so make some noise as you approach blind turns.

The trail makes a swooping right-hander and then sidles up alongside Grabtown Gulch crick. This creekbed is a beautiful cacophony of terrestrial intention, with the life of the creek flowing beneath crisscrossed, mossy fallen trees, ferns, and the dark, living soil. You might be bombing too fast down this trail to really appreciate the visuals, but if you can force yourself, take a moment to stop and enjoy.

After 220 yards along the creek, the trail makes a sharp left, crossing the gulch on a gray-green, high-modulus plastic bridge, which was installed in 2004 after the original bridge was washed out by the 1998 El Niño tropical storm. Following the bridge the trail shrinks in width to just a foot wide and weaves a wicked path around a multitude of redwood trees and then goes around a sharp right-hand switchback before dropping you onto Purisima Creek Trail.

You need to make a sharp left onto Purisima Creek Trail so that you're heading west, which, if you came down that last part of Grabtown Gulch with any speed at all, will necessitate stopping and turning around. However, there is a bridge just up ahead in the wrong direction, and as it is so incredibly beautiful in the creek basin—infused with that fabulous organic smell of a vibrant forest community—you might just want to head over to the bridge and stop for a moment to soak it all in.

Purisima Creek Trail runs along—you guessed it—Purisima Creek. From Grabtown Gulch, head west on Purisima Creek Trail just 110 yards and make a left at the fork onto Borden Hatch Mill Trail.

Borden Hatch Mill Trail is an old logging road that's cut into the hillside and gains in 2.7 miles the elevation that Grabtown Gulch dropped in 1.5. This trail is equally fun, if a bit less hair-raising, to descend as Grabtown Gulch, but because it's easier to climb and because it tends to be popular with hikers, it is generally chosen for the ascent.

This trail winds elaborately up the hill with a fairly consistent gradient. You can tell that it was constructed with the old diesel logging trucks in mind because rather than flow up and down with the contours of the hill, the builders just went with a deeper cut into the hillside to keep the grade consistent. There have been improvements to the trail, some of which are water cuts that, when descending this trail, make for nice jumps.

There are many old, green moss–covered stumps sitting in among the approximately 40-to-70-year-old redwood growth and one or two giant logs that got chopped down but for some reason or other didn't make the truck out back in the logging days (at least one of these looks to be about the size of a truck itself and was maybe just too big to take). This is a great conversational trail, so if you just pick a nice low gear and find a rhythm, you can cruise your way up, checking out the amazing scenery and holding a conversation with your riding partners without getting too out of breath. There are one or two kickers, usually on the back of the water cuts, and a couple of rocky sections, but overall the trail is smooth. Toward the top the Bald Knob hiking trail splits off right, and you're only a half mile from the car, so if you wanted to drop the bikes off in the car and make the 3.6-mile round-trip hike up to the knob, it's completely possible. Make a right at the next fork and then you're backtracking to the car. Take this 0.3 miles to enjoy the smell of the quiet forest while you still can before you head back to whatever urban center it is you call home.

After the Ride

Head over to La Casita Chilanga in Redwood City. This is a great, traditional Mexican food restaurant, and they serve huaraches! Take Tunitas Creek Road up to Skyline Boulevard but pass through it and proceed onto Kings Mountain, which winds through Huddart County Park (no bikes here). Turn left when you reach Woodside Road and then take it 4.5 miles to El Camino Real and turn left. La Casita Chilanga is 1.3 miles north of Woodside Road at 761 El Camino Real (phone (650) 364-2808).

31

KEY AT-A-GLANCE INFORMATION

Length: 5.91 miles

Configuration: Counterclockwise loop

Difficulty: 9/10; just a half mile longer and this loop would get a 10/10.

Scenery: Healthy, young redwood forest and classic California chaparral

Exposure: Rare. Trees cover much of the ride; only Manzanita Trail has any considerable sunlight.

Ride traffic: One of the more accessible loops in one of the most popular parks in the Bay Area for riding, this loop garners a lot of traffic.

Riding time: 1.5–2.5 hours

Access: Free parking for up to 40 cars. Park closes half an hour after sunset.

Facilities: None

GPS TRAILHEAD COORDINATES (WGS 84)

UTM Zone 10S
Easting 0561670
Northing 4139930
Latitude N 37° 24' 21.7"
Longitude W 122° 18' 11.2"

EL CORTE DE MADERA CREEK OPEN SPACE PRESERVE: SHOOTS AND LADDERS

In Brief

This loop gets its name from the wide-eyed combination of descents down Fir and Manzanita trails mixed with the relatively mundane climbs up Methuselah and Timberview trails, respectively. This is the mountain bike park that all other parks should aspire to, and this is the loop where locally based mountain bike R&D folk come to work their trade.

Contact

El Corte de Madera Creek Open Space Preserve
Midpeninsula Regional Open Space District
330 Distel Circle
Los Altos, CA 94022-1404
(650) 691-1200
www.openspace.org/preserves/pr_ecdm.asp

Description

Tip: For this ride, air down your tires 5 to 10 psi lower than normal.

El Corte de Madera Creek Open Space Preserve is jam-packed with trails, 98 percent of which are mountain bike legal, which makes this a very popular place among Bay Area mountain bikers. This ride starts from gate CM02 in the northeast corner of the park, and it is one of the more popular launching points.

DIRECTIONS

From San Francisco, head approximately 13 miles South on Interstate 280 until you come to CA 92/San Mateo Road. Exit CA 92 toward Half Moon Bay. Cross over the Crystal Springs Reservoir and drive 2 miles until you come to the intersection with CA 35/Skyline Boulevard. Turn left onto Skyline Boulevard and drive 8 miles south, through the intersection with Kings Mountain Road, until you see the signs for El Corte de Madera Creek Open Space Preserve.

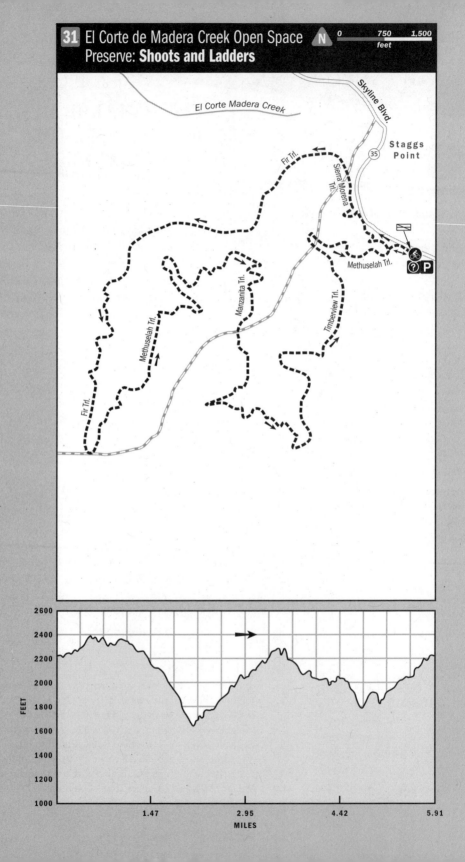

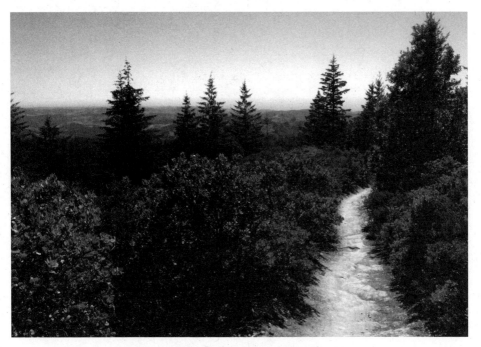

Manzanita Trail takes you out into the sun.

Enter the gate from the parking area along the side of the road, and you're faced with a large signboard replete with a blown-up trail map behind glass, pertinent warnings against the local dangerous flora and fauna, and an endless supply of trail maps.

From the signboard head right. The trail descends quickly before immediately coming to a fork. Go right onto Sierra Morena Trail, a great singletrack that skirts Skyline Boulevard. From the starting elevation of 2,200 feet, Sierra Morena Trail climbs up to the ride's maximum elevation of 2,390 feet in the first quarter mile, before the descending starts.

Along the sides of the trail, you'll notice that many riders have taken to riding on the various irregularities, turning them into makeshift tabletop jumps. Park officials have cracked down on the more impacting of these brief-but-illegal excursions, placing NO BIKES signs at either end of an offshoot, while leaving some of the presumably more harmless versions alone. Please respect the park and stay on the known trails; this is not a true terrain park, and it's a shame to see so many signs going up against the forested backdrop to control our behavior; it reflects poorly on our community.

Sierra Morena Trail meets Fir Trail a half mile into the ride, where it peaks on a small climb. Go left on Fir Trail where it makes a sweeping left through an open space between two of the highest peaks in the park, riding from the west face of one peak to the east face of the other and back into the trees. There is an old, dead, woodpecker-riddled tree standing in a ravine to the left. Within the next 110 yards, you come to the next fork. Go right, continuing on Fir Trail.

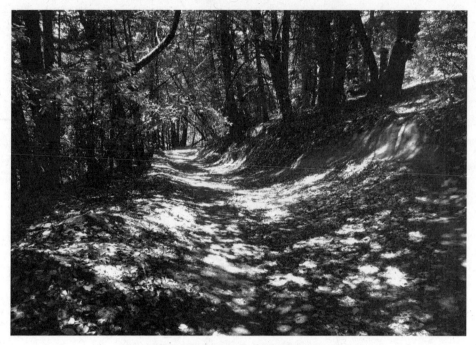

Fir Trail has a few wall-rides like this one.

Initially Fir Trail is an innocuous, rolling doubletrack featuring just a few suspension-awakening, chewed-up spots mixed in with a couple of wall-ride sections that park officials have kindly left open for our enjoyment. Stay on Fir Trail through the next intersection, where Tafoni Trail intersects from the right. Following this intersection there is a steep, rutted, and rocky section.

Make two consecutive lefts at the next two intersections, continuing down Fir Trail. Past the last intersection is where the trail really gets steep. First up is a steep, rocky section that requires you to drop your backside over the seat and hope you don't hit a rock wrong and topple end over end. The trail levels out briefly, running first through some manzanita bushes and then some pine trees where pinecones cover the ground in fall. Then the trail drops again, this time down a very different kind of descent. This is one of the most exciting descents in the Bay Area. Very steep and surrounded by dense foliage, the trail has a slight concave profile and is covered in madrona leaves, making for a slick passage. This trail is the mountain bike equivalent of going down a waterslide. There are also two turns hidden in this deluge of dirt, leaves, and gravity that just beg to be overshot, and signs indicate that it happens regularly. When descending this trail, keep in mind the posted 15 mph speed limit and a heads-up for traffic.

At the bottom of the descent, Fir Trail makes a somewhat precarious junction with Methuselah Trail. Go left on Methuselah Trail, which starts climbing right away. This is the lowest elevation point of the ride at 1,600 feet, and you will be climbing all the way back up to 2,250 in the next 1.4 miles, so if you're not a climber type, you'll need a life span like that of Noah's relative to make it up this climb.

Methuselah Trail is a dusty fire road that climbs up through the redwoods. It's not too technical, although some of the churned up, dusty sections can be difficult to navigate. The park has laid down gravel in sections to help prevent the service vehicles from causing too much damage to the trail. The gravel does help mitigate some of the nefarious traction situations caused by the deep silt, that is unless you forgot to air down your tires 10–15 psi before heading out on this ride. Otherwise you will be skittering all over the gravel. The climbing goes on forever, but once you reach the coyote brush, you're almost at the top.

At mile 3.5 Methuselah Trail connects with Manzanita Trail. You can continue on Methuselah Trail back to the parking lot, but if you're ready for another great technical loop, then turn right onto Manzanita Trail and descend down a pristine singletrack that winds through giant bay and madrona trees, goes through two tight switchbacks, and then pops you out of the trees and into said manzanita bushes, some classic California chaparral, and rocks; this trail has some serious texture to it! Descend a 44-yard, mildly steep, rocky section straight into an almost identical uphill section, both of which are very difficult to ride—it's trials type stuff. The trail continues in this vein for the next 0.3 miles, in the midst of which you actually get some good extended views to the west if you can peel you eyes off the rocks long enough to look.

Manzanita Trail concludes with a smooth singletrack downhill before meeting Timberview Trail at mile 4.5. Make a left onto Timberview Trail, and another left just 0.1 mile on to stay on Timberview Trail, which descends all the way down to 1,800 feet before beginning its climb back up to Skyline Boulevard.

The climb up Timberview Trail feels very similar to Methuselah Trail, and when you find that trail again at mile 5.4, make a right, and you're close enough to let the sounds of the cars on Skyline Boulevard guide you back to the parking lot, all covered in sweat.

After the Ride

Head back into the city and over to Puerto Alegre Restaurant in the Mission District. It's at 546 Valencia Street and you should expect to wait about an hour before you can sit down and enjoy their Milanesa and some tasty margaritas. Bring some energy bars and enjoy the culture on the street as you wait for your table (phone (415) 255-8201).

EL CORTE DE MADERA CREEK OPEN SPACE PRESERVE: BEAR GULCH LOOP

KEY AT-A-GLANCE INFORMATION

Length: 6.79 miles

Configuration: Clockwise loop with 0.1-mile out-and-back

Difficulty: 8/10; not quite as technical as the other ride in this park, but slightly longer and with 15 percent more climbing and descending

Scenery: Mystical redwood forest interspersed with many stumps from the old-growth forest that once was

Exposure: Rare. Trees cover 95 percent of this loop.

Ride traffic: Medium. Not many people choose to enter the park from this access point, but the closer you get to the center of the park, the more people you'll see.

Riding time: 2–3.5 hours

Access: Free parking on Bear Gulch Road, but space for only about 4 cars. Park closes half an hour after sunset.

Facilities: None

In Brief

There are more than 35 miles of trails in El Corte de Madera Creek Open Space Preserve and this is a great, not-too-technical loop in the slightly quieter southeast corner of the park. It ends on Spring Board Trail, which is more of a roller coaster than, well, a springboard.

Contact

El Corte de Madera Creek Open Space Preserve
Midpeninsula Regional Open Space District
330 Distel Circle
Los Altos, CA 94022-1404
(650) 691-1200
www.openspace.org/preserves/pr_ecdm.asp

Description

This loop starts at gate CM06 off Bear Gulch Road, deep in the woods. The woods are quiet out here, but as you get out of the car on a weekend day, you might hear some strains of Shakespeare emanating from the Theatre in the Woods, which is located just another few hundred

DIRECTIONS

From San Francisco, head approximately 13 miles South on Interstate 280 until you come to CA 92/San Mateo Road. Exit CA 92 toward Half Moon Bay. Cross over the Crystal Springs Reservoir and drive 2 miles until you come to the intersection with CA 35/Skyline Boulevard. Turn left onto Skyline Boulevard and drive 10 miles south. Turn right onto Bear Gulch Road. This is a one-lane road, so drive slowly and beware of oncoming traffic. In just under a mile, you'll come to a fork with Allen Road. Continue right on Bear Gulch Road; the small parking lot is on the right-hand side of the road about 75 yards past Allen Road. The park gate is another 15 yards beyond that, somewhat hidden from the parking lot behind a large redwood tree.

GPS TRAILHEAD COORDINATES (WGS 84)

UTM Zone 10S
Easting 0562240
Northing 4137920
Latitude N 37° 23' 16.5"
Longitude W 122° 17' 48.4"

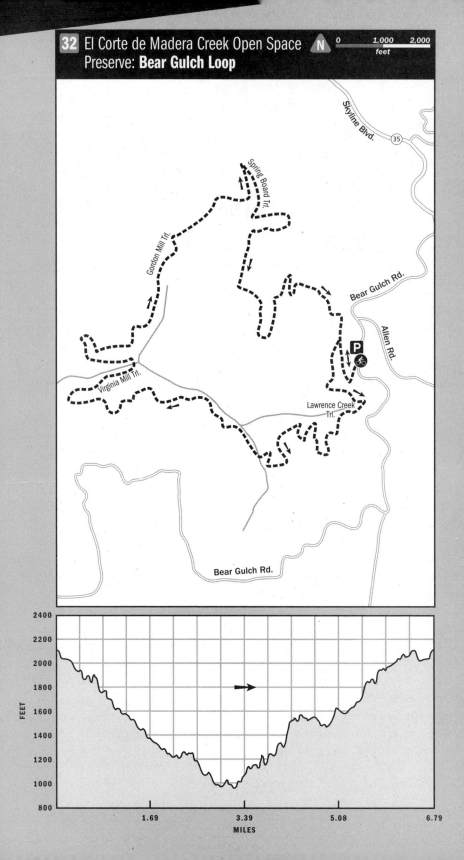

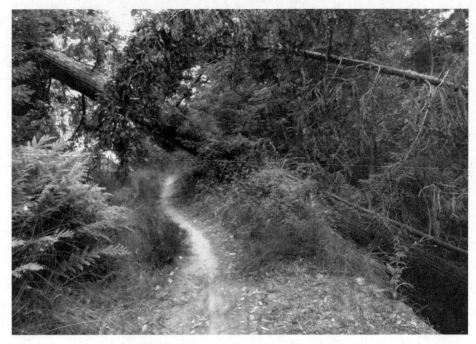

A fallen tree lies across Spring Board Trail.

yards down the road. Hop over the gate and onto Lawrence Creek Trail, which takes off downhill into the woods.

The bulk of the trails in this corner of the park are reappropriated logging roads from the more than a century span of time this area was logged, beginning in the 1860s, and Lawrence Creek Trail is no different. Although effectively a singletrack, this trail sits in a broad cut into the hillside that certainly wasn't made by hooves, boots, or knobbies.

The first intersection comes quickly, and as you make a left, be careful because the trail surface here is very chewed up and there are hidden ruts underneath the deep sand; be careful not to let your front wheel wash out. Continue down Lawrence Creek Trail through the intermixed redwood and evergreen forest.

Blue Blossom Trail appears out of the next clearing of the trees, and the dirt in this intersection is especially white, such that when the sun hits it just right, it can be blinding. When you make the left onto Lawrence Creek and slip back into the woods, you can find yourself a little snow-blind for the first few yards until your eyes adjust.

For the next 0.75 miles, the trail drops down some mild whoop-de-dos with the hillside on the left, makes a sweeping right-hand turn, and then cuts the other way down the hillside. Lawrence Creek generates in a spring in this vicinity and gets steadily more pronounced as it picks up (condensed) steam toward the bottom of the hill.

One of the odd distinguishing factors of this southeast section of the park is the prevalence of off-camber turns, and by some geographic anomaly, they're all left-handers.

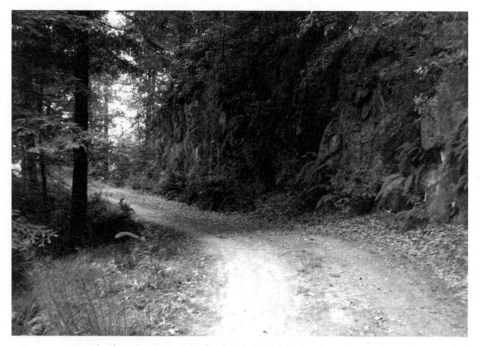

**Roads don't get cut into bedrock like this for recreation alone:
the timber industry greatly shaped this park.**

As you progress down the hill, closer to the basin of the ravine, you begin to see more ferns and lush, water-dependent greenery. At 2.7 miles in, make a right onto Virginia Mill Trail. Some ruts hidden in the lush foliage overgrowing the trail make the transition rough. In the next half mile, the trail makes two consecutive steep drops that bring you down to creek level, 1,200 feet below your starting elevation. Cross the bridge where two springs converge into one and start the climb back up on the other side.

Climbing the first 220 yards out of the creek bed is a difficult task and the last 20-yard pitch takes you up a rutted singletrack surrounded by berry vines. You may have to step off if you lose momentum. At the top Virginia Mill Trail makes a T with Gordon Mill Trail at mile 3.3. Make a right onto Gordon Mill Trail, a doubletrack running up one of those old logging cuts, much like Lawrence Creek Trail. There are a few sections climbing up 10–12 percent grades through here, so be sure to bring your 32-tooth cog, and maybe some of those shocks with lockout. Heck, maybe just bring your hardtail, since unlike other areas of the park, this loop doesn't necessarily require copious suspension travel.

After climbing for 1.2 miles, you'll make a right onto Spring Board Trail. There's a trail sign here, in case you forgot your map and fear you might be lost. Spring Board Trail descends smoothly for about 30 yards to the next fork, where you'll make another right in order to stay on Spring Board Trail (left turn is Steam Donkey Trail). Continue to descend slightly, over a roller that makes for a nice jump, and under a huge fallen redwood tree. Past this there is a steep 45-yard section into a loose left-hander. Then you immediately start climbing again. Once you settle into the climb and things quiet down around you, you'll probably start hearing strange noises emanating from a stream passing through a culvert. The noises change throughout the year, relative to aggregation of water, and by some combination of construction and the natural echo-quality of the ravine, it can sound very different from what it actually is—sometimes like a snarl, sometimes like a large beast walking through the brush—and this makes for a bit of a surprise for someone not expecting to hear it. Past this impressionist culvert, the trail goes up a steep 55-yard climb, at the top of which is a fork.

Make a left at this fork, staying on Spring Board Trail (right is Blue Blossom Trail). Spring Board Trail climbs steadily up through the serene, soft light of the redwood forest. There are many huge old stumps visible among the fairly young redwood growth, indicative of a time when this beautiful space represented nothing more to someone than a cash crop.

Go right at the next fork, continuing on Spring Board Trail as it makes the steepest single descent in the park: a 100-foot drop in about 45 yards. It's a rush, and at the bottom you find yourself back at the chewed-up intersection with Lawrence Creek Trail. The big challenge is being able to stop, or at least properly direct, your motion at the bottom of this descent without allowing the ruts and deep silt to swipe your wheels out from under you. After you dust yourself off, just make a left and head back up Lawrence Creek Trail to gate CM06.

After the Ride

Drive back up to San Francisco and go eat at Shangri La—possibly the best vegetarian Chinese food you'll ever eat. They're located at 2026 Irving Street, between 21st and 22nd avenues in the Outer Sunset district. The items in red on the menu are customer favorites, and the pie pa tofu balls with broccoli will become an addiction, which might be a bit troubling for those of you who don't live in the area (phone (415) 731-2548).

33

KEY AT-A-GLANCE INFORMATION

Length: 2.55 miles

Configuration: Loop with 0.6-mile out-and-back

Difficulty: 1/10; a really simple but fun loop with minor elevation change

Scenery: Classic, oak-studded Northern California rolling hills. There is a vibrant wildlife population in this park; you'll likely see a number of animals, particularly of the winged variety.

Exposure: Moderate

Ride traffic: Heavy on weekends, moderate on weekday afternoons and evenings

Riding time: 0.5–1 hour

Access: No-fee parking in a large, 30-car parking lot

Facilities: Full restrooms and drinking fountains

GPS TRAILHEAD COORDINATES (WGS 84)

UTM Zone   10S
Easting   0573186
Northing   4137944
Latitude   N 37° 23' 13.96"
Longitude   W 122° 10' 24.02"

PEARSON ARASTRADERO PRESERVE: ACORN TRAIL LOOP

In Brief

A great place to bring young kids or anyone who is fairly new to the sport. The terrain is not very demanding and the beauty of the shallow, grassy, oak-studded hills makes for pleasant slow-speed travel with many stops. Acorn Trail at the far end of the loop is the technical and visual highlight of the ride.

Contact

Pearson Arastradero Preserve

1530 Arastradero Road

Palo Alto, CA 94303

(650) 329-2423

www.city.palo-alto.ca.us (click DEPARTMENTS, then COMMUNITY SERVICES, then OPEN SPACE AND PARKS)

Description

The Enid W. Pearson Arastradero Preserve is a beautiful 622-acre park maintained by the city of Palo Alto. This loop is the only nonpaved loop with year-round access. The city maintains a wealth of information on the park, including up-to-date information on seasonal trail closures, all of which can be found both online and on the bulletin board in the parking lot. The sign also gives fair warning that the park lies in typical mountain-lion habitat. There have been no reported attacks on humans, although there have been sightings as well as horses

DIRECTIONS

From San Francisco, drive approximately 30 miles south on Interstate 280 toward San Jose. Take the Page Mill Road exit and turn right (heading west) toward Portola Valley. Drive 0.25 miles, take the first right onto Arastradero Road, and drive 0.3 miles to the parking lot on your right.

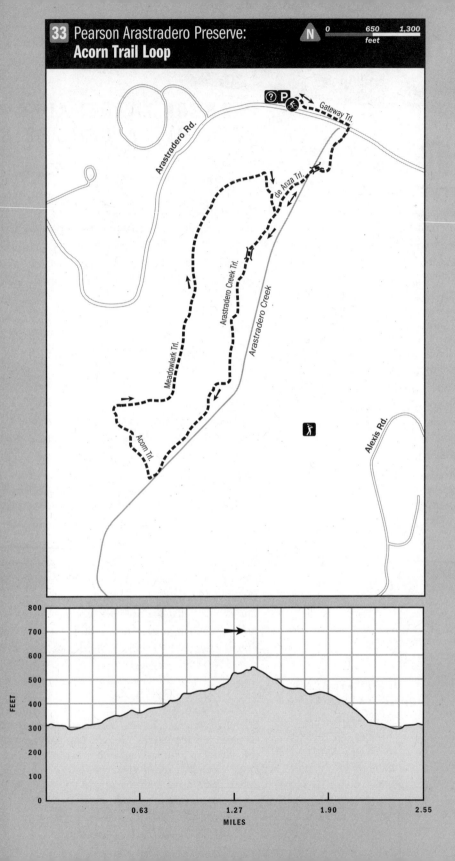

33 Pearson Arastradero Preserve: Acorn Trail Loop

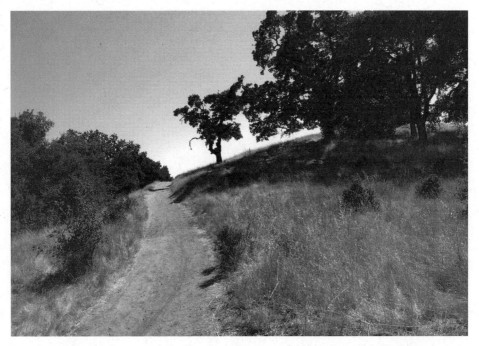

Arastradero Creek Trail going over one of the park's mild climbs

bearing injuries believed to have been inflicted by mountain lions. All in all, the park is safe, but do take the precaution of riding with a partner if possible.

Recently the city built a new restroom facility at the east end of the park, and it has to be one of the most magnificent park restrooms ever built. From the park sign, take the gravel path leading toward the restrooms, bypassing them and continuing on Gateway Trail, which turns right and crosses Arastradero Road at a crosswalk. On the other side of the road, cross Arastradero Creek on a short bridge, pass through Gate A, and then make a right at the first fork onto Juan Bautista de Anza (de Anza) Trail. The signage in the park is plentiful, indicating both the names of the trails as well as where they lead to, so you don't need to worry about winding up at an unmarked intersection if you get off course.

Roll along the smooth doubletrack through the savanna grassland and make a left at the next fork, staying on de Anza Trail. The trail ascends ever so slightly through this section passing bushes of scrub oak and deerweed. You'll probably frighten more than a couple of quail out of the bushes, and they'll run along the trail from one bushy hideout to another. Alone in the middle of one of the grassy fields there is the stump of an old oak tree that looks like it died and rotted away from the top down. The remaining stump looks like a rearing horse's head.

The next fork features a bridge. Make a right, continuing on de Anza Trail. In this area listen for a pair of hawks calling who have built a nest in one of the trees. According to one local bird-watching couple, the hawks' names are Mick and Angie. Through the oak trees and underbrush here you can see Arastradero Lake, which offers year-round fishing.

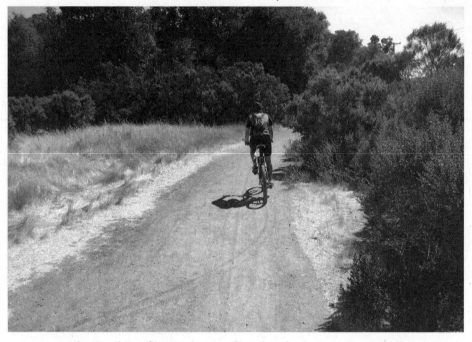

Chaparral is a favorite home of quail and other small animals.

At the next junction, turn left onto Arastradero Creek Trail, a smooth gravel road that follows the creek. Ride past a fenced-in water works facility sporting some bright blue pipes.

It's 0.75 miles to the next fork, a section of trail ramps up a little bit steeper than the rest of the climb. At the peak of the climb is a turn with an old wood fence on the inside. The fence could be there to keep people out of the massive poison oak bushes that clutter the small hillside. Looking straight ahead from this point, about 1 or 2 miles in the distance, a very large house that somewhat resembles an old castle is framed by the nearby trees.

The trail continues to follow the creek, although often hidden behind a wall of dense vegetation growing along the banks. There is a lot of life in these dark woods; take a moment to stop and peer in and catch a glimpse of a garter snake or other reptiles living among the moist berry vines, spreading rush, and red willow trees.

Exactly 1 mile from the parking lot, make a sharp right onto Acorn Trail, which is a great little singletrack that shoots up over a grassy knoll before disappearing into the forest. The climb has about a 5 percent grade, so really young riders might need a little coaxing to get up this little hill.

Acorn Trail levels as it enters an area of oak trees and twists its way out to the other side, leaving you on the open hillside looking down on Arastradero Creek Trail. There are clumps of poison oak bushes dotting the grassy hillside between you and the trail you just left; when the leaves begin to turn red in the fall, they create splashes of color contrasting with the canvas of yellow grass. From this vantage point you can see across to the Palo Alto Hills Golf and Country Club.

The trail dips back into the trees on a slight descent. On a sunny day, the sun streams through the canopy in hundreds of parallel shafts, cutting through the shade of the forest. Next, cross over a puncheon, climb for about 200 feet, and then crest at the highest point of the ride at 550 feet. The views from here are nearly 360 degrees and quite beautiful. At the next fork, turn right onto Meadowlark Trail and enjoy a nice mellow downhill through wide open grassland. There are a few rollers, off which it's possible to catch a bit of air if you try.

Meadowlark Trail comes to a junction with the Juan Bautista de Anza fire road again; head straight through, continuing downhill on the Meadowlark Trail singletrack. At the next fork, where Portola Pasture Trail joins Meadowlark Trail, make a right, continuing on the latter trail. From there the trail veers right a little and then drops sharply for what is the steepest and most technical 300-foot section of descent. The difficulty is due to ruts and a slightly off-camber left-hand turn.

Immediately after that downhill section, the loop completes as Meadowlark Trail meets the de Anza Trail that you rode up earlier. Make a left back onto this trail and backtrack to the parking lot.

After the Ride

Hit up Pizz'a Chicago in Palo Alto. Not only is it probably the best pizza in the valley, but the name is also a linguistic delight for word lovers. Just get back on Page Mill Road and head west, passing under the freeway and continuing until you come to the next major intersection, which is El Camino Real. Turn right and head about a quarter mile to 4115 El Camino Real and get yourself a piece of Pizz'a Chicago's pizza in your favorite flavor (phone (650) 424-9400).

34

Length: 4.78 miles

Configuration: Out-and-back

Difficulty: 4/10; steep climb into a headwind on a choppy trail

Scenery: Ridgeline views down into Portola Valley and out to the coast on a clear day

Exposure: Burnt; a few hiding spots out of the wind and sun, but otherwise wide open

Ride traffic: Heavy on weekends, moderately heavy on weekdays afternoon/evenings

Riding time: 0.75–1.25 hours

Access: Ample free parking around the intersection of Willowbrook Drive and Alpine Road

Facilities: None

GPS TRAILHEAD COORDINATES (WGS 84)

UTM Zone 10S
Easting 0569484
Northing 4135442
Latitude N 37° 21' 53.6"
Longitude W 122° 12' 55.2"

WINDY HILL OPEN SPACE PRESERVE: WINDY HILL OUT-AND-BACK

In Brief

Windy Hill is an aptly named park in Portola Valley, as it is very much wind-blown and very much a hill. The wind does calm down, and when it's not pushing a great amount of fog into the valley, the views can be really beautiful. In fact, just seeing the fog speed over the lip of the ridge is a pretty amazing sight in and of itself; however, particularly heavy fog can settle on certain parts of the trail and affect sight to some degree, so beware on foggy downhills. Bicycle access is limited to Spring Ridge Trail, which is a challenging climb for those interested in a good workout and a fun descent.

Contact

Windy Hill Open Space Preserve
Part of the Midpeninsula Regional Open Space District
330 Distel Circle
Los Altos, CA 94022-1404
(650) 691-1200
http://www.openspace.org/preserves/pr_windy_hill.asp

Description

Starting from gate WH06 on Alpine Road, just around the corner from Willowbrook Drive, the trail cants slightly down toward a bridge. Cross the bridge and make a left onto Meadow Trail. The right-hand option is a private drive, and there are plenty of signs that direct park users

DIRECTIONS

From San Francisco, head approximately 30 miles south on Interstate 280 toward San Jose and take the Alpine Road exit toward Portola Valley. Drive 3.8 miles on Alpine Road to where it intersects with Willowbrook Drive. Park on either Willowbrook Drive or Alpine Road.

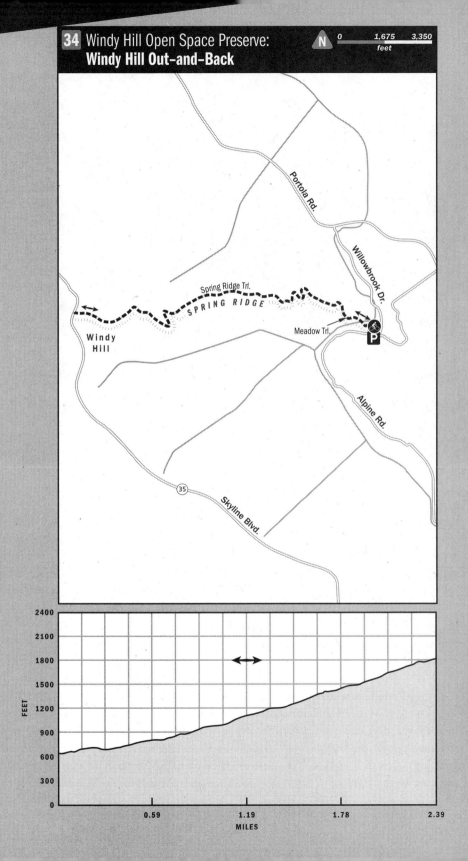

N

0	1,675	3,350

feet

Portola Rd.

Willowbrook Dr.

Spring Ridge Trl.

SPRING RIDGE

Meadow Trl.

P

Windy Hill

Alpine Rd.

35

Skyline Blvd.

FEET				
2400				
2100				
1800				
1500				
1200				
900				
600				
300				
0				

0.59	1.19	1.78	2.39

MILES

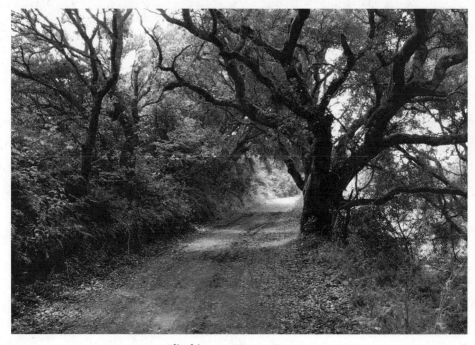

Climbing up Havey Canyon

to stay on the trails and not travel on the driveway. Honestly, though, why would you want to ride up a driveway when you have a fun, twisty little singletrack such as Meadow Trail to warm your legs up on?

The trail climbs up and comes to a fork beneath a large oak tree. Go right at the fork and cross over the private drive, where the trail turns into doubletrack. Ride up this winding doubletrack for 0.6 miles and come to the next fork where you turn left onto Spring Ridge Trail and the trail pitches up steeply and gets rough. The soil in this area is the type that expands a great deal when saturated and shrinks again as it dries, so the trail can be thick and muddy when wet and cracked and pitted when dry.

Stay straight at the next fork, continuing on Spring Ridge Trail. As you pass through a small grove of bay and small madrona trees, the trail turns into a narrow fire road and beyond the trees, there are great views off to the right, with the hillside on your left. It is a stair-step climb, alternating virtually flat sections with quite steep sections that get the lactic acid burning in your legs.

You progress up three protracted switchbacks that take you up through the trees, and then you go around a broad right-hander, the trees open, and suddenly you are on the ridge. At this point you become well acquainted with the park's first name as the wind roars across the ridgetop. If you're in the park in the dry season, as you hit the steep part of the climb, you'll notice that the surface looks wrinkled—almost like you're riding on the back of a great big elephant. Rainwater has run down the face of this climb in bunches of rivulets and then the earth dried out, accentuating each one so that they look like this. Some of

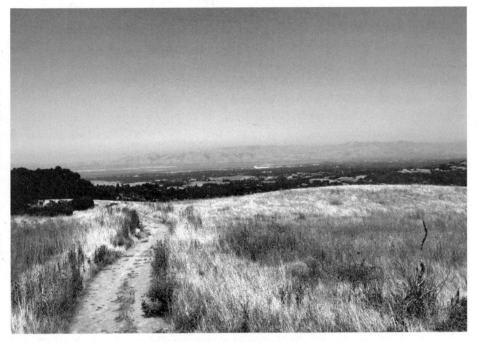

Looking down the hill into Portola Valley

the deeper grooves can redirect your wheel almost as well as a trolley track, so watch yourself, particularly on the descent back down.

At the top of the second steep section, the trail tucks in behind a wall of trees and you get some respite from the up-to-25-mph winds. The trail turns left and levels out, staying hidden from the wind in the cut of the hillside. From here, fog permitting, the views down into Portola Valley can be excellent. Along the ridge to your right is a beautiful array of wildflowers, like the purple owl's clover and morning glories and even some California poppies. You can also see a majority of the trail that you've just come up as it cuts its way up through the rolling grassy hillsides that expand ever outward, spotted with live oaks and chaparral.

Go round the next right-hand bend, and the peacefulness of those hillsides is forgotten. Suddenly it feels like you've wound up in the exhaust of a jet engine while the trail points skyward again. This one section of trail truly calls upon one's powers of Zen thinking: just keep repeating to yourself, "The wind is a beautiful thing, the hills are beautiful things, the burning sensations in my legs and lungs are beautiful things," and it will get you through to the next left-hand turn and back into the safety of the trees.

This is a beautiful, lush area full of poison oak and wildflowers, including rayless arnica, which, if you're handy in the art of processing homeopathic remedies from live plants, you might be able to turn into something to alleviate the pains your muscles are probably feeling at this point in time. There is a small stream running through here, which is causing all of this vegetation to be so happy compared to the rest of the landscape, but it does soggy up the trail a little bit.

The climb persists until the trees grow tired again and the trail spits you out in the open 100 yards before you reach the end of the Spring Ridge Trail where it intersects Skyline Boulevard (Route 35). From here it's just a short walk (sorry, no bikes) up to Windy Hill peak at 1,800 feet, which is 1,200 feet higher than where you started. It's worth pushing the bikes the 0.4 miles up the hiking trail to get 360-degree views, with sightlines all the way out to the ocean. The surrounding hills are covered in dense forest, including many redwood tracts that lead into the other major parks of the region such as Russian Ridge Open Space and the famed El Corte de Madera Open Space. It's a great place for a snack and a stretch before the descent back down to the car.

The park can be really busy, especially on the weekends, so it's not a great idea to attack the downhill with reckless abandon. However, a good way to gauge your speed on the way back down the hill is to remember that you will see a lot of the people you passed on your way up. Also remember: you'll have that crazy wind at your back, acting like blasts of nitrous as it pushes you along.

After the Ride

Hop on Alpine Road heading east back toward town. Pass under the freeway and make a right onto Sand Hill Road, taking this past the Stanford Shopping Center. Make a left onto El Camino Real and drive down to the Santa Cruz Avenue intersection. At 1090 El Camino Real in Menlo Park you'll find the British Bankers Club, affectionately known as the "BBC" to Stanford's beer-drinking elite. It features a fine selection of beers and other assorted drinks plus an attractively priced menu with everything from salmon tacos to an excellent meatloaf. Outside there's a large patio with space heaters for evening meals (phone (650) 327-8769).

COAL CREEK OPEN SPACE PRESERVE: DOG BONE LOOP

KEY AT-A-GLANCE INFORMATION

Length: 4.79 miles

Configuration: Dog bone

Difficulty: 6/10. Moderately challenging technical sections combined with 1,300 feet of climbing and descending equals good fun.

Scenery: Lush forest and incredible bird's-eye views of Palo Alto and surrounding hamlets

Exposure: Rare. Trees do a great job of providing shade here.

Ride traffic: Minimal

Riding time: 1.75–2.25 hours

Access: Free parking

Facilities: None

In Brief

Quasi-hidden relative to the other parks in the Mid-peninsula Regional Open Space District, Coal Creek features fantastic singletrack and one or two stupendous views. If you combine this ride with a ride in neighboring Russian Ridge, you'll get two very different experiences: Coal Creek will make you feel like a forest gnome and Russian Ridge, a grassland-scouring falcon.

Contact

Coal Creek Open Space Preserve

Midpeninsula Regional Open Space District

330 Distel Circle

Los Altos, CA 94022-1404

(650) 691-1200

www.openspace.org/preserves/pr_coal_creek.asp

Description

You can spend time in the parking lot checking out the view of the valley from your 2,334-foot high perch, but really you should just hop on the bike and get on with the ride, because there is a much more scenic vantage point in store for those with a bit of adventure in their legs.

DIRECTIONS

From San Francisco, drive approximately 24 miles south on Interstate 280 until you come to CA 84/Woodside Road. Exit Woodside Road west, toward Woodside. Drive 6 miles on Woodside Road to where it intersects CA 35/Skyline Boulevard. Turn left onto Skyline Boulevard and head south for 7 miles. Just past Clouds Rest Road (on the left, easy to miss), there will be a long swath of paved, roadside parking (also on the left, hard to miss) overlooking the valley floor. This is a popular sightseeing spot—look for folks with binoculars. If you come to the intersection with Alpine and Page Mill roads, you've gone too far.

GPS TRAILHEAD COORDINATES (WGS 84)

UTM Zone   10S
Easting   0570598
Northing   4130975
Latitude   N 37° 19' 28.6"
Longitude   W 122° 12' 11.5"

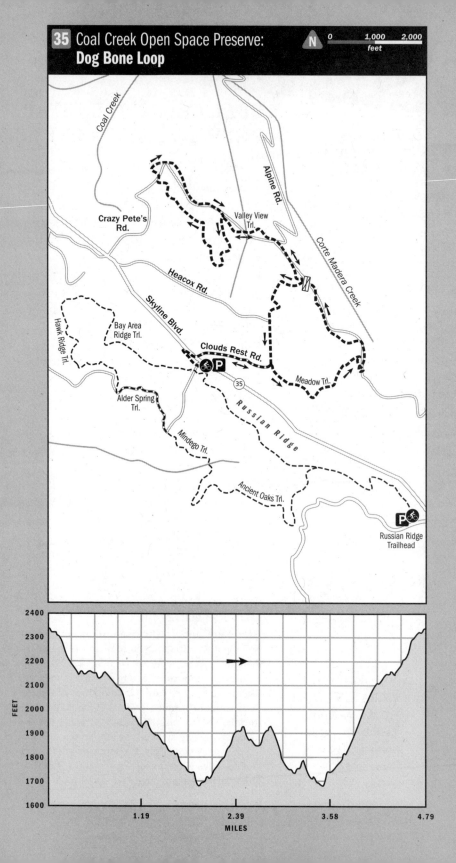

N

0   1,000   2,000
      feet

Coal Creek

Alpine Rd.

Crazy Pete's
Rd.

Valley View
Trl.

Corte Madera Creek

Heacox Rd.

Skyline Blvd.

Bay Area
Ridge Trl.

Hawk Ridge Trl.

Clouds Rest Rd.

35

Meadow Trl.

Alder Spring
Trl.

Mindego Trl.

Russian Ridge

Ancient Oaks Trl.

Russian Ridge
Trailhead

FEET

2400
2300
2200
2100
2000
1900
1800
1700
1600

1.19   2.39   3.58   4.79

MILES

Ride about 300 yards north up Skyline Boulevard to Clouds Rest Road and turn right. Clouds Rest Road is indicated on the park map as Clouds Rest *Trail*, which could explain its condition: full of potholes and loose gravel. Descend on down, passing by the two private drives on the left, and come to gate CO003. The gate is metal, and there is a pedestrian opening along the left side, but there are two logs across the bottom of this opening, necessitating a dismount and portage maneuver.

The poor pavement ends just the other side of the gate, and 220 yards down, you come to an intersection. Turn right onto Meadow Trail, a double-track, which immediately climbs 40 feet up into the woods, surrounded by a lot of poison oak, before leveling out and turning into a ripping singletrack downhill. This is a half-mile descent that takes you out into the open chaparral and then back into the

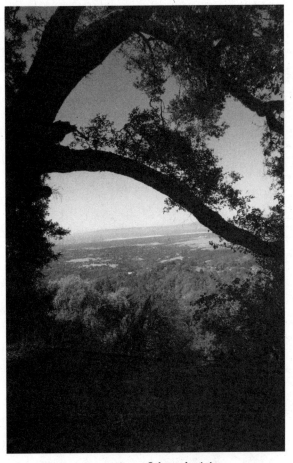

Nature's version of the television set

woods, where you'll go through a tight switchback and bomb down the last 110-yard stretch to Alpine Road. There is a fence at this junction, but it's wide open and easy to ride through. There is a trail sign here with a blown-up map to help you get your bearings.

This section of Alpine Road is dirt and no longer open to cars—hooray! Head down this shady, sometimes narrow road/trail, being sure to watch the mild ruts that run the length. Through the trees to the east, you can catch glimpses of Woodside, but really this trail is about the maples, bays, alders, ferns, oaks, and poison oak that hang over the trail providing shade and color.

At 1.6 miles you come to a fork. Note this fork as you make a right, because you will be coming back to it later. Continue down Alpine Road; from here the trail whips around a blind left-hander, just after which is a washout that might be fixed before the coming wet season. Just 0.2 miles later, you come to the next fork, and here you'll abandon Alpine Road and make a left onto Valley View Trail. This junction is the lowest point of the ride at

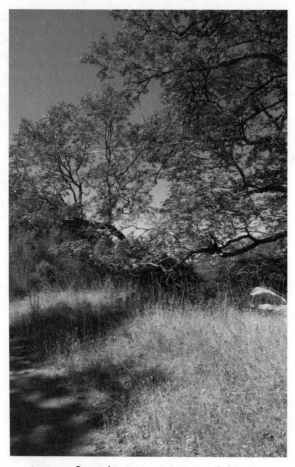

A scene from the Crazy Pete's Road descent

an elevation of 1,730 feet, which means you've descended a total of 600 feet from your car.

Valley View Trail breaks up the rhythm a little bit by popping a quick climb and then making you dismount to hop over an unfriendly series of three logs placed to prevent wheeled egress through the gate placed there. However, remounting the bike is like throwing a leg over the trail itself. This tight, twisty single-track cuts through dense, gorgeous foliage that seems to part for your front wheel. Immediately you cross over a small bridge that takes you over a fantastic little gorge and then you climb slightly up for the next 0.3 miles. The great thing about this ride is that you'll get to experience this excellent chunk of trail in both directions.

Next up you come to Nature's version of a roundabout, where instead of a basic Y intersection, the trails connect in three different spots, encircling a small clump of live oaks. Head left (south) at this junction and remember—you're in the woods, so there're no laws that say you have to take the long way round this roundabout. Start climbing up the narrow dirt road. The trail is fairly steep, averaging a 10.5 percent grade, and it feels like a doozy, especially since you've just spent so much time descending. There are a handful of little singletracks that meet the trail on the left as you climb up; these are just private footpaths that lead up to the nice homes surrounding the park, some of which are visible from the trail.

The payoff for this climb comes at mile 2.4, 1,916 feet of elevation. At this point the trail has gradually turned right and begun to head north, so the downhill is now on your right. What comes into view as you reach the top of this climb is a giant live oak, perfectly shaped to frame the most amazing, scenic view down to the valley floor. The hillside peels away so sharply below the tree that you can almost lose perspective, and the image streams into the shaded trail like TV in a dark living room. Walk up to the oak and look down over the populous valley floor—you feel like you're riding high in a zeppelin with a glass floor. This is truly an irresistible sight and you *will* stop to take it in, even if you're the most die-hard, never-stop-pedaling kind of rider.

Following the lookout, the trail spends another half mile up on this ridge, going through a brief down, then up, before coming to the intersection with Crazy Pete's Road. Make a right and continue on the Valley View Loop, descending back down through the trees to the natural roundabout. The top of this wide singletrack descent is very steep, but it levels out near the bottom, and the trail surface is smooth.

From the roundabout, backtrack to Alpine Road and up Alpine Road to the intersection mentioned earlier. Here you have a choice: you can take the route prescribed here and make the steep uphill, right-hand, off-camber turn up to gate CO002, which will take you up a steep, exposed climb back to gate CO003. Not only will this difficult climb build character, but it will give you the satisfaction of doing the double loop. Perhaps the more enjoyable and sensible thing to do, though, is skip this turn and ride back up the way you came down, enjoying that great early singletrack in reverse. Just a thought.

After the Ride

Head into Google territory (Mountain View) to Mi Pueblo, located at 40 South Rengstorff Avenue. This is actually a Mexican Carniceria and grocery, but they have a to-go window outside where you can grub on some delicious, cheap, authentic Mexican food. There isn't much in the way of tables or chairs, but Rengstorff Park is nearby, so take your tacos and burritos over there and relax on the lawn (phone (650) 967-3630).

36

KEY AT-A-GLANCE INFORMATION

Length: 5 miles

Configuration: Clockwise loop with half-mile out-and-back

Difficulty: 4/10. Total climbing on this loop is only 1,211 feet, and it's fairly well distributed, which means that your legs won't explode.

Scenery: Ridgetop panoramic views with a bird's-eye view of Stanford campus

Exposure: Well-done; bring sunscreen

Ride traffic: Medium. With many good trail options in the area, even nice weekend days aren't too crowded here.

Riding time: 1.75–3 hours

Access: Free parking

Facilities: Restroom, no water

GPS TRAILHEAD COORDINATES (WGS 84)

UTM Zone 10S
Easting 0571980
Northing 4129970
Latitude N 37° 18' 55.7"
Longitude W 122° 11' 15.5"

RUSSIAN RIDGE OPEN SPACE PRESERVE: ANCIENT OAKS TRAIL TO HAWK TRAIL LOOP

In Brief

Part of the extensive Midpeninsula Regional Open Space District, Russian Ridge features a modestly sized and mildly challenging trail network. This ride is the largest complete loop you can do in the park, but there are many offshoots, and there are trails that connect to other parks in this system. The trail network is intelligently laid out, making best use of the steep terrain so as not to have trails that point straight up and down.

Contact

Russian Ridge Open Space Preserve
Midpeninsula Regional Open Space District
330 Distel Circle
Los Altos, CA 94022-1404
(650) 691-1200
www.openspace.org/preserves/pr_russian_ridge.asp

Description

In the parking lot, you'll find an informative trail sign that also offers free maps. The maps are large and detail all eight parks in the South Skyline Region of the Midpeninsula Open Space District. It's a cumbersome map—not the best thing to take out on the trail. If you want a map, it's best to download and print up the Russian Ridge map from the park's Web site.

DIRECTIONS

From San Francisco, drive approximately 24 miles south on Interstate 280 until you come to CA 84/Woodside Road. Exit Woodside Road west, toward Woodside. Drive 6 miles on Woodside Road to where it intersects CA 35/Skyline Boulevard. Turn left onto Skyline Boulevard, head south for just over 7 miles, and make a right onto Alpine Road. The parking lot is about 15 yards from Skyline Boulevard on the north side of Alpine Road.

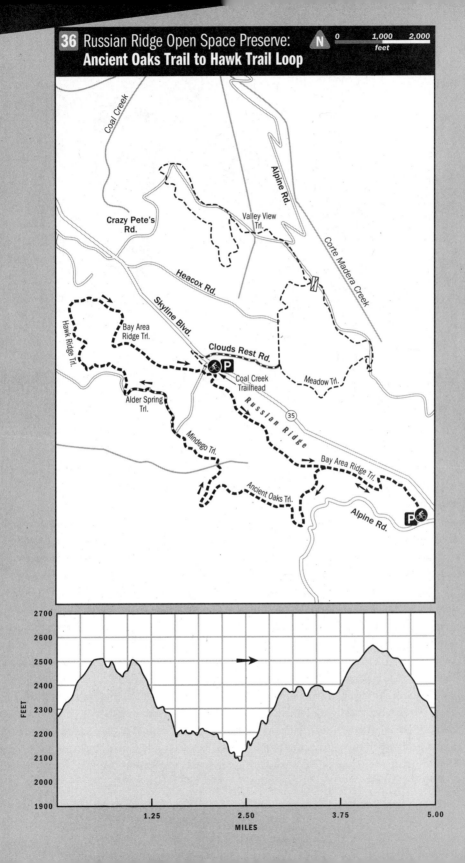

N

0   1,000   2,000
feet

Coal Creek

Alpine Rd.

Crazy Pete's Rd.

Valley View Trl.

Corte Madera Creek

Heacox Rd.

Skyline Blvd.

Bay Area Ridge Trl.

Hawk Ridge Trl.

Clouds Rest Rd.

Coal Creek Trailhead

Meadow Trl.

Alder Spring Trl.

Russian Ridge

35

Mindego Trl.

Bay Area Ridge Trl.

Ancient Oaks Trl.

Alpine Rd.

2700
2600
2500
2400
2300
2200
2100
2000
1900

FEET

1.25   2.50   3.75   5.00
MILES

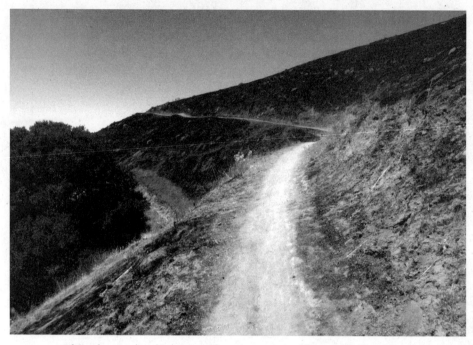

This photo was shot soon after the summer '07 controlled burn.

Starting from the trail sign, head right onto Bay Area Ridge Trail, which is often called just "Ridge Trail" on many of the signs within the park. This is a doubletrack set in the grassy hillsides. It's a half mile to the first junction, and in this space, you'll pass under a stand of buckeye trees and go through an S-curve before you wind up on top of the ridge where the trail widens into a fire road.

At the first intersection, make a left onto Ancient Oaks Trail, which is a level fire road that skirts to the left of the ridge. The first 110 yards of the trail go through more open grassland, and there are views down the hill to Alpine Road and further afield to the south. The trail then descends slightly through a small forest of large live oaks, bay trees, and buckeye trees.

In 0.3 miles, you come to the next fork and make a right onto Ancient Oaks Trail, a singletrack that bounds over a grassy knoll and onto the side of the adjacent hill. In spring this wide-open hillside is smattered with a variety of wildflowers, but in summer it looks like Scrooge McDuck's big mound of gold. There are a few clusters of trees on the hill below the trail, and many large green patches spread throughout the surrounding hills, but Russian Ridge is primarily about enjoying the sun.

There is, however, one big grove of giant oak trees for which this trail is named. You enter the woods on a slight descent, so keep an eye out for the fork that lies just inside the trees. Make a left at the fork, staying on Ancient Oaks Trail. This is a cantankerous old forest made up of primarily oaks and live oaks, but with a few madronas and pine trees thrown in. Some of these old oaks have many trunks sprouting from a common burl,

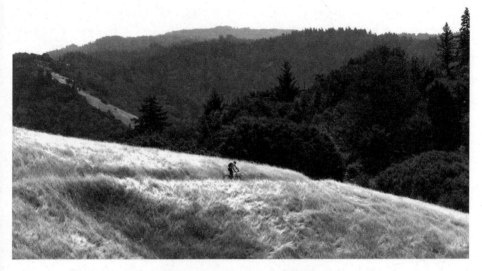

Descending a golden hillside

and these look like giant green hands breaching through the ground. Many of the trees have lightly worn areas where obviously many have been unable to resist the temptation to climb.

The trail through the woods is singletrack. It's not terribly technical but just twisty enough to be interesting, and there are a few exposed roots and mild rocky sections, so you need to keep a keen watch on what you're rolling over. The trail descends through the entire tree section, gradually shrinking into a tiny singletrack. It runs through a particularly lush part of the forest full of ferns and other thirsty plants, indicating that there is an aquifer in the area.

The trail drops down onto Mindego Trail, a fire road onto which you'll turn right. Just 110 yards into this smooth, level trail, you'll pass round a left-hand bend and over the stream that was predicted by the abundant plant life. One stoic old pine tree dominates the area, whilst two of his comrades have gone the way of the woodpecker.

Within 0.3 miles, the trees abandon the trail and your melatonin resumes its vitamin D uptake. Just before the 2-mile mark, you come to the next junction. Make a left onto Alder Spring Trail. In July of 2007, park officials undertook a controlled burn in the northern section of the park, and this intersection served as the southern boundary of the burn. It was quite a sight to see the standard yellow hills juxtaposed against the sooty black sections, very much like an abstracted yin-yang symbol. Park officials posted pictures taken after the burn on the Russian Ridge Web site.

If you were interested in cutting the ride approximately 1.3 miles shorter, you could make the right turn and climb up onto the ridge, taking Ridge Trail south back to the parking lot.

Alder Trail is a wide fire road, and essentially flat, as it continues to the left, running under some large trees and wrapping around the point of the ridge before slipping back into the trees where it begins to descend a bit. And yes, there is a spring that feeds quite a few alder trees, in case you were wondering how this trail might have earned its name.

The most difficult segment of this loop, Hawk Trail, is a singletrack that splits right off Alder Spring fire road at mile 2.4 and begins clawing its way precariously along the steep hillside. You'll climb 280 feet in just a half mile, so be ready to work. With the recent burn, the hillside, with its exposed boulders, takes on an otherworldly aspect. From here you get views all the way out to the ocean near San Gregorio on clear days. The climb gets a little steeper toward the top where it meets up with Bay Area Ridge Trail again at mile 3.

Turn right onto Bay Area Ridge Trail heading south toward Vista Point parking lot. At this point you're fully on top of the ridge with requisite views all around, unobstructed on the treeless hilltop. You can even catch a glimpse of Hoover Tower down on Stanford's campus. The trail runs right along the top of the ridge, which is more or less flat and about as wide as a soccer field. At first the trail favors the western side of the ridge and then switches over to the right.

At mile 3.7 you come to the junction with Clouds Rest Trail. Clouds Rest Trail cuts west over Skyline Boulevard and into Coal Creek Open Space Preserve. If you're looking to extend your ride, this is a great way to add an extra loop, and that loop is described on page 191. Cut straight through this intersection, continuing on Ridge Trail, which kicks up over a small climb at the top of which is a great lookout point—the highest spot on this ride. From here it's practically a no-brainer to get back to the car, just head straight through the next two intersections and backtrack the last half mile through the S-curve and under the buckeye trees.

After the Ride

For your burrito fix after the ride, head over to Mextogo in Menlo Park, just up the road from Stanford. Located at 1081 El Camino Real, this place is both oddly named and oddly delicious (phone (650) 321-9669).

KEY AT-A-GLANCE INFORMATION

Length: 8.48 miles

Configuration: Counterclockwise loop

Difficulty: 7/10; a long ride, but not exceedingly technical

Scenery: Shady creek-bed ecosystems, pine and oak forests (when crossing the creek be thoughtful of the impact)

Exposure: Medium-rare. First two-thirds of the ride are completely covered, while the last third features some extended sunny sections.

Ride traffic: Low. Because of its length, Canyon Trail doesn't see very high traffic numbers.

Riding time: 2.5–4 hours

Access: Free parking. Park is open sunrise to sunset.

Facilities: In the parking lot of the Skyline Ridge Open Space Preserve, halfway through the ride, you'll find water and restrooms.

GPS TRAILHEAD COORDINATES (WGS 84)

UTM Zone 10S
Easting 0575040
Northing 4127240
Latitude N 37° 17' 26.3"
Longitude W 122° 9' 11.7"

SOUTH SKYLINE REGION OPEN SPACE PRESERVE: FOUR PARKS LOOP

In Brief

This large loop takes you on a survey of four of the parks that line Skyline Boulevard: Upper Stevens Creek County Park, Monte Bello Open Space Preserve, Skyline Ridge Open Space Preserve, and Long Ridge Open Space Preserve. This is one of the biggest contiguous loops on offer in the area, and it's relatively smooth and unencumbered with technically demanding sections, so it won't leave you too thrashed at the end.

Contact

Midpeninsula Regional Open Space District
330 Distel Circle
Los Altos, CA 94022-1404
(650) 691-1200
www.openspace.org/preserves/maps/south_skyline_map_07-04.pdf

Description

This ride begins with a 1,000-foot drop from Skyline Boulevard at 2,300 feet elevation down to Stevens Creek at 1,350 feet elevation, but you have a choice as to what size "parachute" you use to get down; from Skyline Boulevard, Grizzly Flat splits in two just past the sign at the trailhead, giving two options for the descent. You have the left option, which is like having a parachute sized for

DIRECTIONS

From San Francisco, drive approximately 24 miles south on Interstate 280 until you come to CA 84/Woodside Road. Exit Woodside Road west, toward Woodside. Drive 6 miles on Woodside Road to where it intersects CA 35/Skyline Boulevard. Turn left onto Skyline Boulevard, head south for 8.9 miles, and look for a long, dirt parking lot on the left of the road.

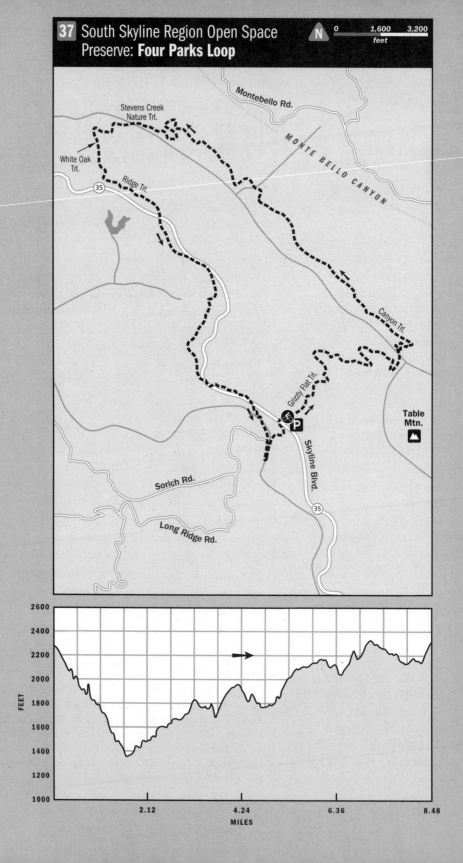

N

0   1,600   3,200
feet

Montebello Rd.

MONTE BELLO CANYON

Stevens Creek
Nature Trl.

White Oak
Trl.

Ridge Trl.

35

Canyon Trl.

Grizzly Flat Trl.

P

Table
Mtn.

Skyline Blvd.

35

Sorich Rd.

Long Ridge Rd.

2600
2400
2200
2000
1800
1600
1400
1200
1000

FEET

2.12   4.24   6.36   8.48

MILES

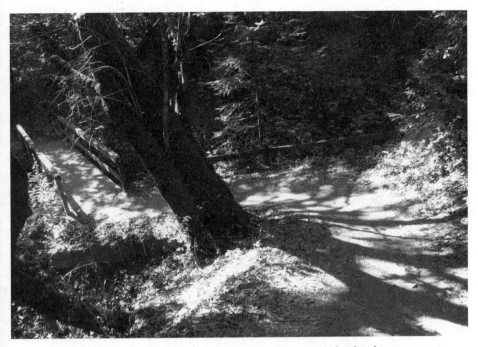

There are multiple crossings of Stevens Creek—some bridged, some not.

someone just a few pounds lighter than yourself, and then you have the right option, which drops like a . . . Led Zeppelin.

Both options are steep, and your humble narrator is advocating taking the left option, North Grizzly Flat, because it is a slightly more *enjoyable* descent. This is an old, narrow dirt road, and although it is wide, there is generally one favored line running down. If you come across another trail user and must leave this line for a moment to pass, just beware that it may be rough and, in fall, provide some surprises beneath the accumulated leaves (nothing that current suspension offerings shouldn't be able to smooth out, though).

There is a turnoff to the right that appears at mile 1.1. Ignore this as it just connects to the south Grizzly Flat option. A few seconds past this is a tight left-hand switchback, the outside of which features the evidence of the many people that have blown through this turn. The steepness of the trail does not belie the steepness of the terrain, and there are some very precarious drop-offs alongside the trail at certain points, but fortunately this one tricky turn is not placed at one such spot.

At mile 1.7 the descent bottoms out and the two Grizzly Trails meet. Make a left onto the singletrack toward Canyon Trail. There is a small, faded trail sign at this junction to give some direction. This tight singletrack runs past a gigantic fir tree before coming into view of Stevens Creek, which it crosses with nary a bridge or a puncheon. Obviously, because of this intimacy with the creek, this trail is not a good pick in the wet season when the creek can swell significantly and present a danger. Also keep in mind, wet season or no, to tread lightly in the creek as even small disturbances can be damaging to this type of ecosystem.

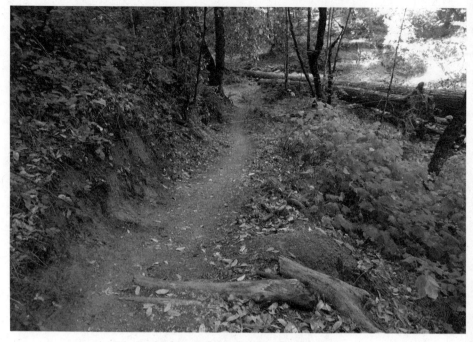

At the base of the Grizzly Flat descent

From the creek the trail climbs 50 feet up a series of six very rapid and tight switchbacks that are reinforced with wood forms and railings. The span between turns is a short 20 to 30 feet, and it feels like you're ascending one of those corkscrew slides from the playground. At the top of this, the singletrack continues to skirt along one of the feeder creeks running perpendicular to Stevens Creek for another 0.12 miles, squeezing through some bay and oak trees before it Ts into Canyon Trail.

Turn left onto Canyon Trail. In an odd bit of civilized wilderness, there are trail signs way out here in the middle of nowhere; one welcoming you to the Monte Bello Open Space Preserve, another reminding cyclists that helmets are required.

Canyon Trail is an old dirt road that rides along the east shore of Stevens Creek roughly 20 to 50 yards above the creek bed. There is nothing too dramatic about the terrain, just a lot of ups and downs, a few small wall rides here and there, and a whole lotta scenic woodland. There are descending mile markers running along this trail, and if you watch these, you'll know that the longest climb comes between mile markers 2 and 1.5. There are also many small singletrack offshoots, some of which loop left to give the rider a better view down into the ravine, and some loop right for the single purpose of veering off the main trail and maybe going over a small jump or two.

When the odometer tics over 4 miles, you come to an intersection. Make a left toward Monte Bello parking (indicated by a trail sign). It's 0.2 miles from this intersection to the next, and that is filled with a quick descent followed by a quick climb, and another descent. Make a left at the junction onto Stevens Creek Nature Trail toward Skyline Boulevard.

Stevens Creek Nature Trail is a ripping-fast singletrack, closed to cyclists and equestrians in the wet season. The trail descends back down to Stevens Creek, passing through a couple of Formula 1–style turns before bottoming out at the creek at 1,830 feet elevation. This time, rather than none, you have three bridges to cross. Of course, since creeks inhabit crevices, once you cross you must do some climbing again. Just 110 yards past the final bridge, you must don your +1 armor and fight the dragon . . . . Not really, but you *will* come to another junction.

Make a left onto White Oak Trail, while Stevens Creek Trail continues to the right as a hiker-only trail. Climb up to the next junction and make another left toward Skyline Boulevard (marked by a trail sign). Ride up a fire road, through an open field past an elegant live oak, and find yourself at Skyline Boulevard.

You've spent 5.4 miles on the dirt, and you have the option here of turning left onto Skyline Boulevard and riding the pavement back to the car. But if you're up for some more dirt—and I know you are—then cross Skyline Boulevard and ride into the Skyline Ridge Open Space Preserve.

Turn left in the parking lot and find Ridge Trail where it begins at the south end of the lot. Ridge Trail (aka The Bay Area Ridge Trail) runs parallel to Skyline Boulevard. Ride this trail for the next 2.6 miles, climbing gradually. There are a couple of good, quick descents thrown in, including a particularly steep and rocky drop at mile 6.7 that immediately slams into an even-steeper and rockier climb, but this 0.3-mile section is an exception on Ridge Trail rather than the rule.

It's easy to follow Ridge Trail, it being the alpha trail in the area—a fire road, sometimes doubletrack, that cuts a determined path southward. There are many offshoot trails competing for your attention, but for the first 1.3 miles, make a series of left turns to avoid getting caught up in the web of trails that make up the Skyline Ridge Preserve. Beyond that there isn't an extensive trail network between Skyline Ridge and Long Ridge parks, with just Ridge Trail diving into the woods and running parallel to Skyline Boulevard. Ignore all offshoot trails, as these are all private driveways.

The next intersection you should be concerned with comes at mile 8; it is here that you will make a 176-degree left-hander onto Peter's Creek Trail. The ride finishes off your aching legs with a half-mile climb, gaining almost 200 feet elevation back up through the trees to Skyline Boulevard and the Grizzly Flat parking lot, making you wish you could somehow MacGuyver that imaginary parachute into a hot-air balloon.

After the Ride

When you get back to your car, head south on CA 35/Skyline Boulevard to CA 9/Big Basin Way, and turn left. Head east on Big Basin Way, driving down out of the hills. When you get back into civilization, make a left onto Saratoga Sunnyvale Avenue, heading north, and drive 2.4 miles. Saratoga Sunnyvale Avenue turns into South de Anza Boulevard, and at 1480 South de Anza Boulevard, you find Layang Layang, a popular Malaysian restaurant. It's a long drive, so you'll probably need to munch on a bar to stave off the hunger pains, but the sizzling beef dish at Layang Layang is well worth the wait (phone (408) 777-8897).

Length: 6.88 miles

Configuration: Clockwise loop with 0.75-mile out-and-back

Difficulty: 8/10. This ride has everything.

Scenery: Panoramic views from 2,500 feet elevation, lovely woods, and a pond

Exposure: Medium-rare; tree cover over much of the ride

Ride traffic: Low

Riding time: 2–3 hours

Access: Free access; parking for about 20 cars at trailhead. Park open sunrise to sunset.

Facilities: None

GPS TRAILHEAD COORDINATES (WGS 84)

UTM Zone 10S
Easting 0576210
Northing 4124900
Latitude N 37° 16' 11.2"
Longitude W 122° 8' 25.4"

LONG RIDGE OPEN SPACE PRESERVE: THE FULL POND LOOP

In Brief

A fantastic loop that features everything from chutelike singletrack descents to exposed fire-road climbs and even a pond. You might couple your visit to this park with a visit to the Jikoji Zen Center (please call ahead (498) 741-9562) for a weekend of self-centering.

Contact

Long Ridge Open Space Preserve
Midpeninsula Regional Open Space District
330 Distel Circle
Los Altos, CA 94022-1404
(650) 691-1200
www.openspace.org/preserves/pr_long_ridge.asp

Description

The trailhead, gate LR01, is located on the west side of Skyline Boulevard. If parked on the east side of the road, be careful crossing because vehicles tend to drive a little too fast for conditions. Pass through the gate and start up the doubletrack, which climbs 220 yards up to a small clearing. Make a right at the clearing and continue climbing.

In another 110 yards, you come to an intersection, and it doesn't matter which direction you choose because

DIRECTIONS

From San Francisco, drive approximately 24 miles south on Interstate 280 until you come to CA 84/Woodside Road. Exit Woodside Road west, toward Woodside. Drive 6 miles on Woodside Road to where it intersects CA 35/Skyline Boulevard. Turn left onto Skyline Boulevard and head south 10.9 miles, at which point you should begin looking for two small pullouts on either side of the road with telltale trail signs. This area is shady and may prevent you from seeing the trailheads. If you come to the Saratoga Summit Fire Station, you've gone 1.5 miles too far.

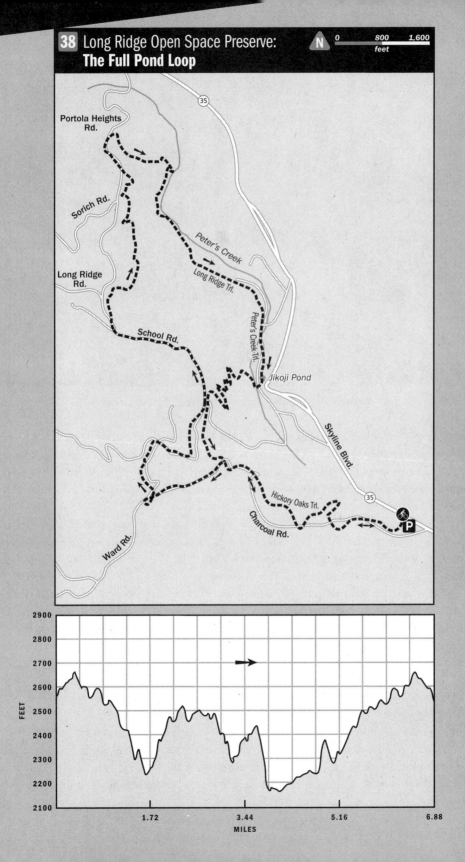

N

0   800   1,600
feet

Portola Heights Rd.

Sorich Rd.

Peter's Creek

Long Ridge Trl.

Long Ridge Rd.

Peter's Creek Trl.

School Rd.

Jikoji Pond

Skyline Blvd.

Hickory Oaks Trl.

Charcoal Rd.

Ward Rd.

P

FEET

2900
2800
2700
2600
2500
2400
2300
2200
2100

1.72   3.44   5.16   6.88

MILES

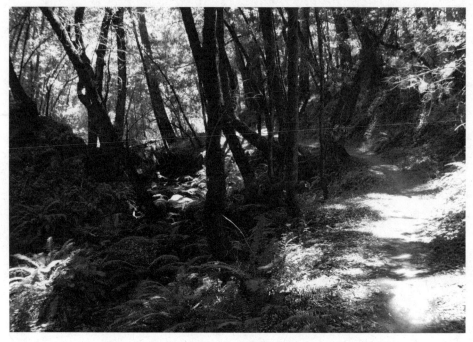

There is a preponderance of ferns in Peters Creek.

they both deposit you onto Hickory Oaks Trail just a short while later. Make a left onto Hickory Oaks and ride out into the open, following as the trail swoops to the left down a slight descent through the grass. There are boulders large and small scattered everywhere and a couple of aptly placed park benches that you may want to plop yourself down on the way back to enjoy some of the long views to the southwest.

Continue descending, and at mile 1.1 you come to the next fork, marked with a sign. Make a left to stay on the Hickory Oaks fire road. Descend for another 0.3 miles (the final tenth of which is very steep) and when the trail passes in between two medium-size live oaks, you'll know that the descent is shortly coming to an end.

Make a sharp right turn onto Ward Road, an old gravel-and-dirt road that initially starts out as level before descending for another 0.2 miles to where it meets School Road. Make a right and stay on Ward Road. Just in case you wondered if these were indeed roads, there are typical green California road signs at the intersection of these two seemingly abandoned dirt roads.

Climbing through the trees, the road is smattered with gravel, which can negatively affect your traction if you've got your tires at a high pressure. In summer that particularly annoying breed of small flies that like to calmly and deliberately assail your face and ears often plague this section. I recommend dousing up with a bit of bug spray for sanity's sake. Pro racers would have a difficult time climbing faster than these little buggers can fly.

At mile 2.1 the climb peaks at the intersection with Long Ridge Road after gaining 200 feet of elevation from the base. Make a left onto Long Ridge Road, a fire road that

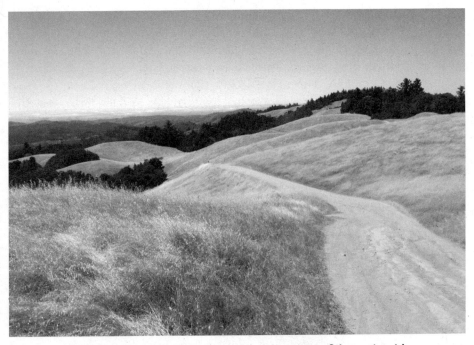

Hickory Oaks Trail is the most exposed portion of the entire ride.

meanders along for another half mile. There are many presumably illegal singletracks peeling off here and there. Many of these have been marked with signs NOT A TRAIL, but others have yet to be marked. They are easily identified by the matted grass on the trail surface, which says that the trail is not maintained. Please stay on marked trails.

Turn right at the next intersection. Going left will just take you to gate LR04 and out to Portola Heights Road. Going right, however, will treat you to one of the more fantastic, ripping, rolling singletracks that Northern California has to offer. The turns on this trail are exquisite. From banked to rocky and technical to tight switchback . . . this trail easily checks all the boxes on the Most Desirable Features of a Trail list. The trail is on a mild decline all through this section. Oh, and there is a cool little gnome's cave hidden in there somewhere, too.

Peter's Creek Trail joins Long Ridge Road from the right at mile 3.2, and Long Ridge Road actually turns into Long Ridge Trail, continuing to the left and passing by gate LR12 about 20 yards later. The trail begins climbing again, goes round a switchback, and then pops out of the woods on a very tight section through some manzanita bushes. From here you can see Portola Heights Road about 40 feet below.

The trail reenters the woods and makes a broad right-hand turn, passing by a private drive, and then takes you down a steep, rough singletrack descent. This is the most technical part of the entire ride, dropping 200 feet in just 0.1 mile. Fortunately, this section is densely shaded, so you don't have to worry about bright sunspots playing with your vision.

At the base of the descent, you find yourself at a lush, fern-laden intersection of creeks. Make a right to stay on Long Ridge Trail, which rides along Steven's Creek. Going left will give you the option of either Bay Area Ridge Trail or Grizzly Flat Trail, in case you're interested in stringing together some of the rides in this book for a truly epic day.

Long Ridge Trail morphs into Peter's Creek Trail and heads south, climbing up out of the woods and through a meadow. The trail has been built up a few inches above the meadow surface with dirt and gravel and lined with small logs to protect both the meadow and the trail. Make a right at the intersection at mile 3.9 and continue climbing up Peter's Creek Trail for another half mile until you come to Jikoji Pond.

This is truly a beautiful little pond owned and maintained by the Jikoji Zen Center, just up the hill. The road to the left of the pond that leads up to the Zen center is gated off, but this is definitely the spot where you want to plan on enjoying your energy bars and maybe snap a few pics with the cell phone, trying to accurately render the ducks that live there.

Cross the dam that runs along the north end of the pond to where Peter's Creek Trail resumes on the other side. This trail is closed in the wet season, so be sure to plan your ride and call ahead or check the Web site for trail closures. Pass through a gate—which will be closed if conditions are too wet—and head up the hill.

From here the trail does a Tazmanian Devil impersonation and climbs up through eight rapid switchbacks. At the top you'll come to a gate, also closed in wet conditions, and just past this is the intersection of Ward and Long Ridge roads, which you should recognize from earlier in the ride. This time around, make a left onto Long Ridge Road and ride 110 yards to the next intersection where you'll make a right and descend down an exposed singletrack that drops you back onto Hickory Oaks Trail. Go left and backtrack to the car.

After the Ride

Call your friend that works at Google and drive on over to the campus in Mountain View to be treated to lunch at Café 150. The concept behind this private restaurant is that they only cook with ingredients obtained within a 150-mile radius of Google, and the food is delicious. (Note you can only get in if you know a Google employee.)

ALMADEN QUICKSILVER COUNTY PARK: MINE HILL AND RANDOL TRAILS LOOP

In Brief

This is a 10-mile romp around the Capitancillos Ridge, which rises up out of a wealthy urban area south of San Jose. Comprised mostly of smooth fire road, this ride isn't going to draw on your technical riding abilities too much, but you are guaranteed to get a good workout. The loop can be conveniently shortened and routed to pass many of the historical quicksilver (mercury) mining sights if, say, you've got your youngsters along. If you're looking for a longer ride, you can connect into neighboring Sierra Azul Open Space Preserve for a serious adventure.

Contact

Almaden Quicksilver County Park

21350 Almaden Road

New Almaden, CA 95042

(408) 323-1107

www.parkhere.org/portal/site/parks

Description

There are only two trailheads that embark from this parking lot: Mine Hill Trail, which starts today's ride and is prominently centered in the parking lot, and Deep Gulch Trail, which is hidden in the southern end of the lot and not open to mountain bikers anyhow. Pass around

GPS TRAILHEAD COORDINATES (WGS 84)

UTM Zone 10S

Easting 0604380

Northing 4114620

Latitude N 37° 10' 27.5"

Longitude W 121° 49' 27.2"

DIRECTIONS

Drive south out of San Francisco 35 miles on CA 101. Exit onto CA 85S/Stevens Creek Freeway and drive south 18 miles. Take the exit toward Almaden Expressway and turn left onto Almaden Plaza Way; drive 300 feet and turn right onto Almaden Expressway. Drive south on Almaden Expressway 4.1 miles and turn right onto Almaden Road. Drive just under 3 miles south and turn right into the parking lot.

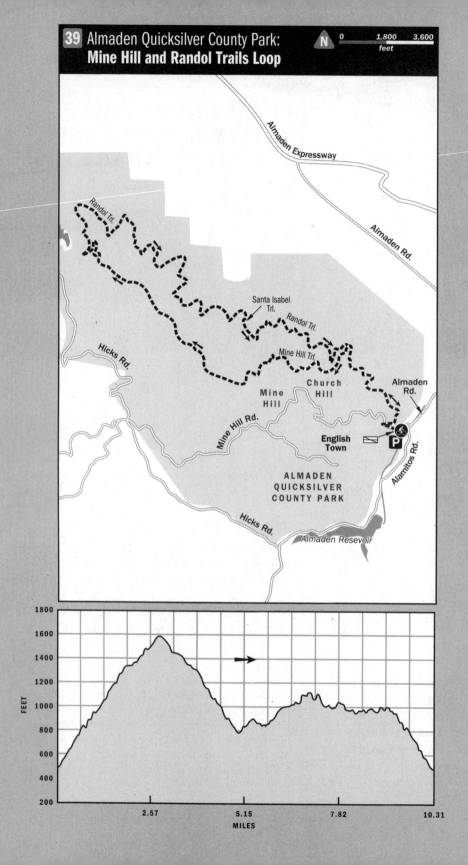

N

0   1,800   3,600
                 feet

Almaden Expressway

Almaden Rd.

Randol Trl.

Santa Isabel
Trl.

Randol Trl.

Mine Hill Trl.

Hicks Rd.

Church
Hill

Almaden
Rd.

Mine
Hill

Mine Hill Rd.

English
Town

Alamitos Rd.

ALMADEN
QUICKSILVER
COUNTY PARK

Hicks Rd.

Almaden Resevoir

FEET

1800
1600
1400
1200
1000
800
600
400
200

2.57   5.15   7.82   10.31

MILES

the gate and start riding up the Mine Hill fire road.

Out of the parking lot the trail immediately gains elevation, and off to the left you get a view of a large field with a small fenced-off portion that contains some large, rusty mining equipment. The fire road is very wide at this point, as it is one of the major arteries in the park, open to all sorts of nonmotorized trail users, including horse carts. This park isn't most advanced in terms of attitude toward mountain bikers (of the 34 total miles of trails, only 10 are open to bikes), but one good policy is that in cases of rain and wet terrain it closes to all, which keeps the pot-marking from horse hooves to a minimum.

Settle into a nice climbing groove because you'll be heading up for the first 3 miles of the ride. You can get an excellent sustained effort out on this climb, since they kept it to a nice 8 percent average grade. If you've got big quads (or just want to hurt

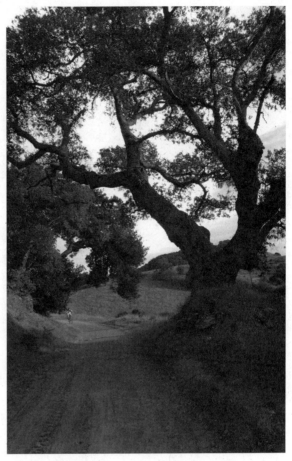

A giant oak frames Mine Hill Trail.

yourself) then jam it in the big ring and alternate between seated and standing to spread the work over the different muscle groups, but if you prefer seated climbing just stick it in the granny gear.

Ignore the first intersection you come to, less than half a mile into the ride, as both the right and left option are no-bikes trails. A mile up the hill you'll come to the next four-way intersection. Make a left to stay on Mine Hill Trail; the middle option is Randol Trail on which you'll be returning later.

On the way up, you're surrounded mostly by live-oak and bay trees, with increasingly elevated views east to the city of New Almaden peaking through here and there. Park wildlife tends to avoid this highly trafficked trail, but you will often see squirrels, maybe deer, and, if you are hawk-eyed, maybe even a bobcat.

Mine Hill Trail makes a sharp right at the next wide-open intersection with Castillero Trail. There is a stone horse trough and tie-post here, and a couple power lines run

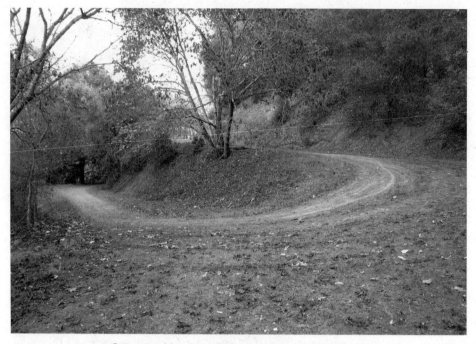

A fast switchback with plenty of room for mistakes

overhead. If you're looking to extend the ride into Sierra Azul Open Space Preserve, then make a left onto Castillero Trail and follow it to where Wood Trail splits off to the left. Follow Wood Trail all the way, across paved Hicks Road and into Sierra Azul. From there, a popular loop is Kennedy Trail (right turn), to paved Kennedy Road (right turn), Shannon Road (right turn), Hicks Road (left turn), Camden Avenue (right turn), and McAbee Road (right turn), at which point you'd follow McAbee Road to its end in Almaden Quicksilver Park and you'd take New Almaden Trail back to the Hacienda entrance. This adds a considerable amount of miles, and pavement, to the ride.

You can make a much smaller loop by taking Castillero Trail and, instead of taking Wood Trail, following Castillero Trail all the way to where it intersects Mine Hill Trail a second time and then taking Mine Hill back to the car. This small loop takes you past four of the park's bike-accessible historical mining sites and is a great loop for kids.

For today's ride, though, avoid Castillero Trail and follow Mine Hill as it continues to climb along the northwestern face of Mine Hill. In the remainder of the climb, you'll pass by April Trail on the right, which is a small little loop that leads out to the Powder House historical site and then reconnects with Mine Hill Trail. The climb taps out at mile 2.9, with a total elevation gain of 1,080 feet from the Hacienda parking lot. Right around this point you'll make a right at the second intersection with Castillero Trail to stay on Mine Hill Trail.

From here the trail descends down the spine of the ridge with commanding views on all sides. You'll pass beneath a gigantic old live oak that forms an arch over the trail.

Then the Guadalupe Reservoir comes into view. On the right kind of cloudy day, the white of the clouds reflects silver off the water and the lake looks like mercury. There actually is a good deal of mercury in the lake, and park users are warned against swimming in the lake or eating the fish caught in it.

The ridge drops off steeply as it approaches the reservoir. The descent here gets twisty to compensate, passing through a couple of broad switchbacks and a third, tighter switchback. Bike-legal Providencia Trail shoots out the back of this final switchback and leads out to a quaint picnic spot overlooking the reservoir. The descent bottoms out at the next intersection, where Mine Hill Trail loses bike status and marches off to the west, leaving you to make a right turn onto Randol Trail fire road, which wraps around the foot of the ridge and begins to head east, back toward Hacienda parking lot.

For the first 2 miles, Randol Trail climbs pretty steadily, dipping in and out of the multiple finger ridges that feed up to the spine of Mine Hill, along which you rode west earlier. The trail is largely exposed, though surrounded by oaks, live oaks, bay trees, and coyote brush, and a bit of poison oak is scattered on the hillsides, but this shouldn't prove a problem from the fire road. Through the trees, in a few spots are good views across the Almaden country clubs and suburbs all the way up to Mount Hamilton. Culverts allow the trail to cross the handful of springs that run down the mountain without issue, and the trail surface is pretty smooth, allowing you to get some leg-buster intervals in without worrying about traction.

Some 2.6 miles into Randol Trail, cyclists must detour onto Santa Isabel Trail, as a 0.7-mile section of Randol Trail is oddly closed to bikes. Santa Isabel Trail offers the same fire-road experience as Randol, but it takes you past the Santa Isabel Mine Shaft. Next to the actual rock-and-mortar remains of the mine is a large info board with graphs and captioned pictures. Opposite the mine are a tangle of rusted cable and pieces of a large old flue, presumably from the mine itself, left for effect by park management. Where this trail Ts back into Randol Trail, be sure to turn right in order to head back to the car.

In the final stretch of Randol Trail, you'll pass by another info board, for the Day Tunnel, a gigantic rusted metal gate (open), and a scenic 25-foot-tall cliffs with ivy and ferns along the face and a couple of prosaic oaks stationed at the top. From there, the Randol Trail terminates at a familiar four-way intersection with Hacienda and Mine Hill trails. Head straight through the intersection and back down the hill to the parking lot on Mine Hill Trail. You'll be tempted to take this descent fast, but be aware that this is the most highly trafficked trail in the park and that the gravel and mild ruts can undermine your ability to stop.

After the Ride

The nearest grub to Almaden Quicksilver park can be found in the Almaden Shopping Center at 5353 Almaden Expressway in San Jose. Here you'll find Mountain Mike's Pizza (phone (408) 268-6630) and Lee's Village Chinese Food (phone (408) 997-7199). If you want to sit down for some delicious enchiladas and a beer, try Tacos Al Pastor—it is a bit pricier than most Mexican restaurants, but the portions make it worth it (phone (408) 997-3548).

40

BIG BASIN REDWOODS STATE PARK: MIDDLE RIDGE AND GAZOS CREEK LOOP

KEY AT-A-GLANCE INFORMATION

Length: 13.69 miles

Configuration: Loop with 1.5-mile out-and-back

Difficulty: 8/10; 3,800 feet of climbing

Scenery: Dense redwood forest, some ancient growth, and a glimpse of the ocean

Exposure: Rare; much of this ride is spent in the eaves of the great redwoods

Ride traffic: Low—too long a loop for most hikers (besides, they have all the singletrack trails they could want)

Riding time: 2–3.5 hours

Access: $6 day-use parking fee, $2 trail map. Campsites are available, but be prepared to book far in advance for a weekend trip.

Facilities: Restrooms, water fountains, and the Big Basin store for essential supplies (closed December and January)

In Brief

At 70 miles distant, this ride is the farthest from San Francisco in this book, but it definitely offers you a drive's worth of mountain biking. Although it's possible to do it as a day trip from the city, to fully enjoy Big Basin you should camp there. A few days in Big Basin will give you time to complete the ride, enjoy the plethora of hiking trails, and, as the park literature suggests, "rediscover the lost art of relaxation," staring up through the branches of the gentle ancient beings. Fortunately, Big Basin isn't one of the state parks on the list of potential closures under Governor Arnold Schwarzenegger's 2008–2009 budget proposal.

Contact

Big Basin Redwoods State Park
21600 Big Basin Way
Boulder Creek, CA 95006
(831) 338-8860
www.parks.ca.gov/default.asp?page_id=540 or
www.bigbasin.org

GPS TRAILHEAD COORDINATES (WGS 84)

UTM Zone 10S
Easting 0569190
Northing 4113570
Latitude N 37° 10' 7.2"
Longitude W 122° 13' 14"

DIRECTIONS

From San Francisco, head south on Interstate 280 toward San Jose. Drive approximately 37 miles on I-280. Take CA 85/Stevens Creek Freeway South toward Gilroy and drive 2.5 miles. Take the De Anza Boulevard exit and turn right onto South De Anza Boulevard, which will become Saratoga Sunnyvale Road. Drive 2.7 miles, then turn right onto Big Basin Way/CA 236 and drive 13.5 curvy miles into the hills. At the next major four-way intersection keep straight, continuing on Big Basin Way for another 8, even more-curvy miles, into the heart of the redwoods. When you come around a great big old redwood, the visitor center will come into view.

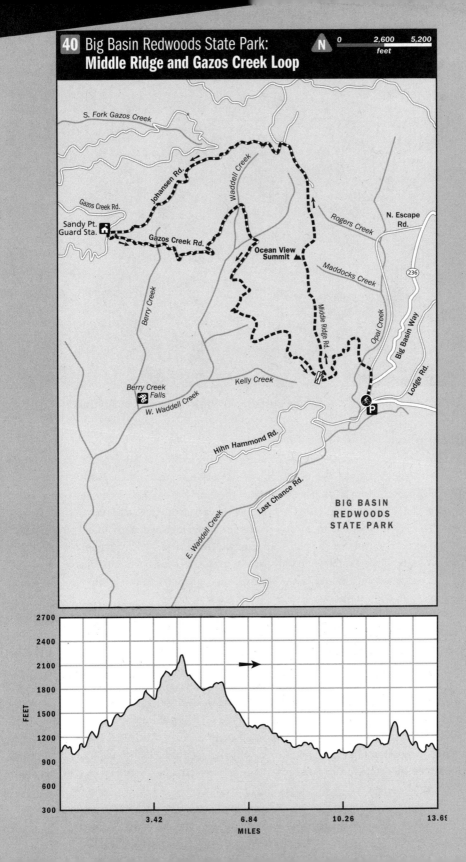

N

0   2,600   5,200
feet

S. Fork Gazos Creek

Johansen Rd.

Waddell Creek

Gazos Creek Rd.

Sandy Pt.
Guard Sta.

Gazos Creek Rd.

Rogers Creek

N. Escape
Rd.

Ocean View
Summit

Maddocks Creek

236

Berry Creek

Middle Ridge Rd.

Opal Creek

Big Basin Way

Lodge Rd.

Kelly Creek

P

Berry Creek
Falls

W. Waddell Creek

Hihn Hammond Rd.

BIG BASIN
REDWOODS
STATE PARK

Last Chance Rd.

E. Waddell Creek

2700
2400
2100
1800
1500
1200
900
600
300

FEET

3.42   6.84   10.26   13.69

MILES

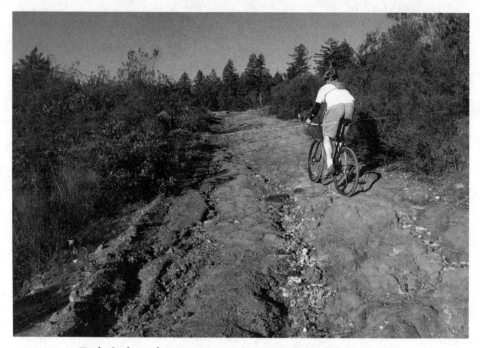

Technical sandstone outcropping near Ocean View Summit

Description

The last 5 miles of the drive into the park are on a primarily one-lane paved road that twists tightly through the trees. When you get to the park headquarters you'll have to check in, whether you're getting a campsite or are just there for the day. Campsite registration must be done inside the main building, but day passes can be purchased at the parking kiosk, if open. The camping situation in California is seriously impacted, particularly on weekends, and it's recommended that you plan your trips well in advance and be prepared to make your campsite reservations right when they become available—yes, a whole *six months* from stay date. If you're not constrained by a Monday–Friday gig and can camp mid-week, you have slightly better odds of finding a site closer to your stay date.

To find the trailhead, turn right at the kiosk onto North Escape Road, and after 310 yards look for an old wooden bridge on the left—this is Gazos Creek Fire Road. You can ride around the usually closed ranger gate on the little footpath to the left and start climbing up the hill.

Pavement persists for the first eighth of a mile up Gazos Creek Road and then turns into the dark rocky soil indicative of the fire roads throughout the park. The fire roads are relatively smooth, with the underlying rocks showing through more heavily in spots; generally, the most technical difficulty you'll experience on this ride is the occasional tree branch lying across the trail. Watch out as you ride over branches on the trail because they can flip up into your spokes and cause some serious damage, especially on descents when momentum is high.

Gazos Creek Road winds up the hill, away from the behemoth redwoods among which the park headquarters are built and up into a much younger forest that has reforested well following the logging that stopped in 1902. You'll pass by a few of the enticing yet illegal singletracks, such as Creeping Forest and Dool Trails, and then, 1.3 miles from the bridge, you'll find your next junction as Middle Ridge Fire Road splits off to the right.

Pass through the gate, beyond which is a burned out redwood with a triangular hole in the base. Middle Ridge Road definitely brings the steep; it's not a gradual climb but spikes and relaxes, even throws in a couple of quick descents. The moist forest floor is home to a wide variety of salamanders, newts, snakes, and other reptilians and amphibians that thrive in such ecology. Sharp-eyed mycologists will delight in the wealth of mushrooms growing up from the decomposing pine needles that form the forest floor and from the moist bark of the trees.

A little over a mile into the Middle Ridge climb, the redwood forest begins to give way to a Douglas fir and chaparral affair, and the surface of the trail gradually turns into more of a sandstone composite, until suddenly you find yourself on a totally exposed patch of trail, scrambling over a bright yellow, heavily textured sandstone wash. This is the most technical stretch of the entire ride, fallen trees notwithstanding.

The exposure, the sandstone, the 1,679-foot elevation . . . it can be none other than Ocean View Summit. If you take a look west, on a clear day you can see the Pacific Ocean shimmering blue at the base of the tree-green valley about 6 miles away as the crow flies. A trail sign points to a small lookout/make-out point just a few feet off the trail. If you see anybody at all on this ride, you're likely to find them there. The spot is a great place for a snack if it's empty.

Past Ocean View Summit, the trail turns right, passes over a sandy wash, reenters the forest, and immediately begins climbing again, to the strains of your voice saying, "Summit, my a#@!" Yes, Virginia, there's more climbing yet. For the next 1.4 miles it's more of the same frenetic, spiky climbs, netting another 600 feet of elevation, to peak out at 2,234 feet (and that's from a starting elevation of 1,007 feet). This peak coincides with the next major trail junction and is marked by an info board that tells of the natural wonders of Berry Creek Ridge, down which you are shortly about to descend. Make a left onto Johansen Fire Road, which is demarcated by one of the ugliest trail signs in existence—a simple white road sign with JOHANSEN RD stenciled on in flat black spray paint. It may be an ugly sign, but its efficiency in communication is highly appreciated this far from camp.

Johansen Fire Road descends down the spine of Berry Creek Ridge. It's fairly straight-forward, except for a couple of the bulldozer turnouts, which at speed can be momentarily confused for the trail itself. The gradient switches positive for a brief bit in the middle of the descent, but it's barely a climb to get worked up about. You may be enticed to stop by the incredible views to the south where you can spot Buzzard's Roost, which is a highly recom-mended hike if you've got a few days to kill in Big Basin. At the bottom of the descent you'll notice a few large, white teepees off to the left, as well as a small log cabin and an old, rusty boxcar on a small section of train track. Don't get too distracted, because the descent ends in a large metal gate.

The teepees and the seemingly misplaced Southern Pacific Lines boxcar are encompassed by an elaborately sculpted metal fence and marked as private. This area is known as Sandy Point. Turn left and follow the fence on the other side of the teepees until you see a sign pointing to Gazos Creek Road (left) and Whitehouse Canyon Road (right); go left.

Gazos Creek Fire Road continues to descend, heading east back along Berry Creek Ridge, passing the namesake stream within the first half mile, and descending gradually down through a redwood, pine, madrona, and bay-tree forest to where it crosses West Waddell Creek, one of the larger creeks in this watershed. At this crossing, the creek cascades over a large expanse of exposed bedrock, passing under the elevated roadway, and turns into a lax waterfall on the downhill side of the trail.

After the creeks, the fire road begins to climb again, after having dropped down to a low elevation of 900 feet. If you left the ride until later in the day, the sun will be fading rapidly on you as you are sunk fairly deep in the redwood forest, just below the westernmost ridges. If you're running without an odometer, you might start wondering how long of a trip you have to get back to camp. The sunset can also be a supremely alluring time in this part of the forest as the last clusters of deep-orange rays of sunlight find their ways through the dense network of trees and illuminate small bits of the forest with the glow of the phoenix.

Right about the time the last of those orange spirits leave the deep forest for favor of the campfires, the climb tops out and you begin descending again just as the forest turns dark and misty and the fact that you left without headlights starts to freak you out. You come to an intersection with Middle Ridge Fire Road and you know you're home at last. Make a left onto Middle Ridge and continue down the hill. Everything should be vaguely familiar at this point, even in the dusk. Pass around the gate and be careful as you ride across the old bridge, because the damp wood picks up moisture fast and is as slick as ice and unwilling to consider the finer functions of cycling, such as turning or braking. Head back to the car or camp and get the grub on.

After the Ride

If you're doing the day-trip thing and are all out of energy bars at the end of the ride but don't want to scarf down cold hot dogs from the Big Basin store, be prepared for the long drive back out of the park. Right before you reach CA 85 on South de Anza Boulevard, you'll find Los Dos Compadres #2 Taqueria on the right side of the road, at 1652 South de Anza Boulevard in San Jose. If the hunger hasn't incapacitated you, sit yourself down and order one of their wet burritos and a beer to replenish your energy stores (phone (408) 777-8805).

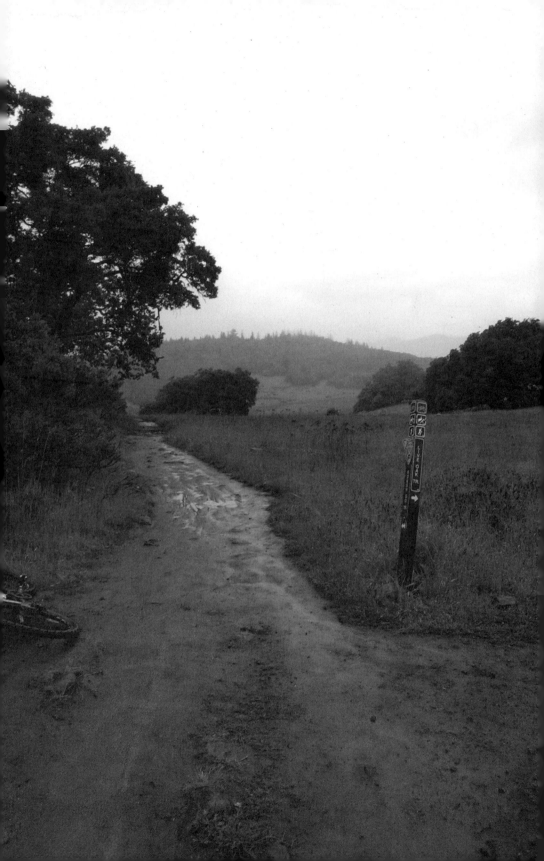

APPENDIXES AND INDEX

APPENDIX A:
Bicycling Clubs in the Greater San Francisco Bay Area

Alto Velo
1785 Balsa Avenue
San Jose, CA 95124
(408) 287-4425
www.altovelo.org

Berkeley Bicycle Club
P.O. Box 165
Berkeley, CA 94701
(510) 527-3222
www.berkeleybike.org

Cal Cycling
University of California, Berkeley
2198 University Avenue
Berkeley, CA
(510) 644-3643
www.calcycling.org

Cherry City Cyclists
P.O. Box 1972
San Leandro, CA 94577
(510) 357-2967
www.cherrycitycyclists.org

Davis Bike Club
610 Third Street
Davis, CA 95616
(530) 756-0186
www.davisbikeclub.org

Different Spokes San Francisco
P.O. Box 14711
San Francisco, CA 94114
(415) 721-4546
www.dssf.org

Eagle Cycling Club
3335 Solano Avenue
Napa, CA 94558
(707) 226-7066
www.eaglecyclingclub.org

Eden Cycling Club
3318 Village Drive
Castro Valley, CA 94546

(510) 881-5000
www.edenbicycles.com

Fremont Freewheelers Bicycle Club
P.O. Box 1868
Fremont, CA 94538
(510) 888-3787
www.fremontfreewheelers.org

Grizzly Peak Cyclists
Membership Chair
377 Oak Park Drive
San Francisco, CA 94131
(510) 482-0912
www.grizzlypeakcyclists.org

East Bay Cyclists
(InfoVista Cycling Team)
841 Tanager Road
Livermore, CA 94551
(925) 606-9975
www.ebcyclist.org

Los Gatos Bicycle Racing Club
c/o Barry Gordon
16230 West Ellenwood Avenue
Monte Sereno, CA 95030-5212
(408) 395-6611
www.lgbrc.org

Marin Cyclists
P.O. Box 2611
San Rafael, CA 94912
(415) 479-8222
www.marincyclists.com

Mountain Bikers of Santa Cruz
P.O. Box 331
Santa Cruz, CA 95061-0331
www.mbosc.org

Norcal Racing
425 College Avenue
Santa Rosa, CA 95401
(707) 573-0112
www.norcalcycling.com

Norcal High School Mountain Bike Race League
4412 Piedmont Avenue #1
Oakland, CA 94611
(510) 653-BIKE
www.norcalmtb.org

Oakland Yellowjackets
2185 Manzanita Drive
Oakland, CA 94611
(510) 986-9011
www.oaklandyellowjackets.org

Peninsula Velo
c/o Randy Smith, 171 Madera Avenue
San Carlos, CA 94070
(415) 345-5616
www.peninsulavelo.org

Responsible Organized Mountain Pedalers (ROMP)
P.O. Box 1723
Campbell, CA 95009-1723
(408) 257-8284
www.romp.org

Rio Strada Racing
P.O. Box 933
Citrus Heights, CA 95611-0933
(916) 442-5246
www.riostradaracing.org

Sacramento Bike Hikers
5470 Grant Avenue
Carmichael, CA 95608
(916) 381-5338
www.bikehikers.com

Sacramento Golden Wheelmen
777 12th Street, Suite 250
Sacramento, CA 95814
(916) 682-0979
Tripp@gfsacto.com
http://sacgwo.tripod.com/pg2002/
    index.html

Sacramento Wheelmen
P.O. Box 15739
Sacramento, CA 95852
(916) 641-2953
www.sacwheelmen.org

San Francisco Bicycle Coalition
995 Market Street
San Francisco, CA 94103
(415) 431-BIKE
www.sfbike.org

San Jose Bicycle Club
(408) 297-5393, www.teamsanjose.org

Santa Cruz County Cycling Club
P.O. Box 8342
Santa Cruz, CA 95061-8342
(831) 689-9580
www.santacruzcycling.org

Santa Rosa Cycling Club
P.O. Box 6008
Santa Rosa, CA 95406
(707) 823-0941
www.srcc.memberlodge.com

Skyline Cycling Club
P.O. Box 60176
Sunnyvale, CA 94088
(408) 736-9858
http://skylinecycling.tripod.com

Team Roaring Mouse
1352 Irving Street
San Francisco, CA 94122
(415) 753-6272
www.teamroaringmouse.com

Team Spine
c/o Kerri Kazala, Manager
901 Campus Drive, Suite 312
Daly City, CA 94015
(650) 755-0859
kerri@spinaldiagnostics.com
www.teamspine.com

Team Wrong Way
teamwrongway@yahoogroups.com
www.teamwrongway.com

Trailworkers.com of Santa Cruz County
www.trailworkers.com

UC Davis Cycling Team
sportclubs.ucdavis.edu/cycling

Valley Spokesmen Bicycle Touring Club
P.O. Box 2630
Dublin, CA 94568
www.valleyspokesmen.org

For a list of all the registered cycling clubs in California, see USA Cycling's Web site:
www.usacycling.org/clubs/
    index.php?state=CA

APPENDIX B:
Bicycling Retailers in the Greater San Francisco Bay Area

San Francisco

American Cyclery
510 Frederick Street
San Francisco, CA
(415) 664-4545
www.americancyclery.com

Avenue Cyclery
756 Stanyan Street
San Francisco, CA 94117
(415) 387-3155
www.avenuecyclery.com

Big Swingin' Cycles
2260 Van Ness Avenue
San Francisco, CA 94109
(415) 441-6294
www.bigswingincycles.com

Bike & Roll
899 Columbus Avenue
San Francisco, CA 94133
(415) 771-8735
www.bikeandroll.com

Bike Doctor
2455 27th Avenue
San Francisco, CA 94116
(415) 759-7431

Bike Hut Foundation
40 Pier
San Francisco, CA 94107
(415) 543-4335
www.thebikehut.com

The Bike Nook
3004 Taraval Street
San Francisco, CA 94116
(415) 731-3838

Bikenut LLC
2221 Filbert Street
San Francisco, CA 94123
(415) 931-0666
www.bikenut.us

Blazing Cycles
1095 Columbus Avenue
San Francisco, CA 94133
(415) 202-8888
www.blazingsaddles.com

Blazing Saddles Bike Rentals
2715 Hyde Street
San Francisco, CA 94109
(415) 202-8888
www.blazingsaddles.com

Box Dog Bikes
494 14th Street
San Francisco, CA 94103
(415) 431-9627
www.boxdogbikes.com

City Cycle of San Francisco
3001 Steiner Street
San Francisco, CA 94123
(415) 346-2242
www.citycycle.com

DD Cycles
4049 Balboa Street
San Francisco, CA 94121
(415) 752-7980
www.ddcycles.com

Freewheel Bike Shop #1
914 Valencia Street
San Francisco, CA 94110
(415) 643-9213
www.thefreewheel.com

Freewheel Bike Shop #2
1920 Hayes Street
San Francisco, CA 94117
(415) 752-9195
www.thefreewheel.com

Fresh Air Bicycles
1943 Divisadero Street
San Francisco, CA 94115
(415) 563-4824

Golden Gate Park Bike
3038 Fulton Stret
San Francisco, CA 94118
(415) 668-1117
www.goldengateparkbikeandskate.com

Heavy Metal Bike Shop
82 29th Street
San Francisco, CA 94110
(415) 643-3929
www.heavymetalbikeshop.com

Lombardi Sports
1600 Jackson Street
San Francisco, CA 94109
(415) 771-0600
www.lombardisports.com

Mike's Bikes of San Francisco
1233 Howard Street
San Francisco, CA 94103
(415) 241-2453
www.mikesbikes.com

Noe Valley Cyclery
4193 24th Street
San Francisco, CA 94114
(415) 647-0886

Nomad Cyclery
2555 Irving Street
San Francisco, CA 94122
(415) 564-3568
www.nomadcyclery.com

Ocean Cyclery
1935 Ocean Avenue
San Francisco, CA 94127
(415) 239-5004
www.oceancyclery.com

Pacific Bicycles
345 Fourth Street
San Francisco, CA 94107
(415) 928-8466
www.pacbikes.com

Pedal Revolution
3085 21st Street
San Francisco, CA 94110
(415) 641-1264
www.pedalrevolution.org

Performance Bike Shop
635 Brannan Street
San Francisco, CA 94107
(415) 856-0230
www.performancebike.com

REI – Recreational Equipment, Inc.
840 Brannan Street
San Francisco, CA 94103
(415) 934-1938
www.rei.com

Road Rage Bicycles
1063 Folsom Street
San Francisco, CA 94103
(415) 255-1351

Roaring Mouse Cycles
1352 Irving Street
San Francisco, CA 94122
(415) 753-6272
www.roaringmousecycles.com

San Francisco Cyclery
672 Stanyan Street
San Francisco, CA 94117
(415) 379-3870
www.sanfranciscocyclery.com

San Francisco State University Campus Bike Barn
600 Holloway Avenue
San Francisco, CA 94132
(415) 338-3170

Sports Basement (Crissy Field)
610 Mason Street
San Francisco, CA 94129
(800) 869-6670
www.sportsbasement.com

Sport Basement (SOMA)
1415 16th Street
San Francisco, CA 94103
(415) 437-0100
www.sportsbasement.com

Valencia Cyclery
1077 Valencia Street
San Francisco, CA 94110
(415) 550-6600
www.valenciacyclery.com

North Bay

Above Category
38 Millwood Street
Mill Valley, CA 94941
(415) 389-5461
www.abovecategory.net

Bici Sport
139 Kentucky Street
Petaluma, CA 94952
(707) 775-4676
www.bicisportusa.com

Bicycle Madness
2500 Jefferson Street
Napa, CA 94558
(707) 253-2453
www.bicyclemadness.com

A Bicycle Odyssey
1417 Bridgeway
Sausalito, CA 94965
(415) 332-3050
www.bicycleodyssey.com

Bicycle Works
3335 Solano Avenue
Napa, CA 94558
(707) 253-7000

Bike Peddler
605 College Avenue
Santa Rosa, CA 95404
(707) 571-2428
www.norcalcycling.com

Bike Rx Depot
231 Flamingo Road
Mill Valley, CA 94941
(415) 407-8960
www.bike-rx.com

Caesar's Cyclery of Marin
29 San Anselmo Avenue
San Anselmo, CA 94960
(415) 721-0805

Cambria Bicycle Outfitters
2885 Santa Rosa Avenue
Santa Rosa, CA 95404
(707) 579-5400
www.cambriabike.com

Cycle Dynamics Bike Shop
5670 Dempsey Place
Santa Rosa, CA 95403
(707) 545-2453

Hub Cyclery
7885 Old Redwood Highway
Cotati, CA 94931
(707) 795-6670
www.thehubcyclery.com

Marin Mountain Bike Wholesale
265 Bel Marin Keys Boulevard
Novato, CA 94949
(415) 382-6000
www.marinbikes.com

Mike's Bikes of San Rafael
1601 Fourth Street
San Rafael, CA 94901
(415) 454-3747
www.mikesbikes.com

Mike's Bikes of Sausalito
1 Gate 6 Road
Sausalito, CA 94965
(415) 332-3200
www.mikesbikes.com

Mill Valley Cycle Works
357 Miller Avenue
Mill Valley, CA 94941
(415) 388-6774
www.millvalleycycleworks.com

Mt. Tam Bikes
244 Shoreline Highway # B
Mill Valley, CA 94941
(415) 389-1900
www.mt.tambikes.com

Napa River Velo
796 Soscol Avenue
Napa, CA 94559
(707) 258-8729
www.naparivervelo.com

Norcal Bike Sport
425 College Avenue
Santa Rosa, CA 95401
(707) 573-0112
www.norcalcycling.com

Paradigm Cycles
702 San Anselmo Avenue
San Anselmo, CA 94960
(415) 454-9534
www.paradigmcycles.com

Performance Bicycle of San Rafael
369 Third Street # A
San Rafael, CA 94901
(415) 454-9063
www.performancebike.com

Petaluma Cyclery
1080 Petaluma Boulevard North
Petaluma, CA 94952
(707) 762-1990

REI – Recreational Equipment, Inc.
213 Corte Madera Town Center
Corte Madera, CA 94925
(415) 927-1938
www.rei.com

REI – Recreational Equipment, Inc.
2715 Santa Rosa Avenue
Santa Rosa, CA 95407
(707) 540-9025
www.rei.com

Rincon Cyclery
4927 Sonoma Highway
Santa Rosa, CA 95409
(707) 538-0868
www.rinconcyclery.com

Road and Tri Sport
366 Bel Marin Keys Boulevard
Novato, CA 94949
(415) 786-9181
www.roadandtrisports.com

Santa Rosa Cyclery
4325 Montgomery Drive
Santa Rosa, CA 95405
(707) 537-2254
www.santarosacyclery.com

Scarfacci Bicycle Company
710 West Napa Street, Suite 3
Sonoma, CA 95476
(707) 938-3753

Sonoma Bicycle Company
264 Petaluma Boulevard North
Petaluma, CA 94952
(707) 776-0606
www.santarosacyclery.com

Sonoma Valley Cyclery
20093 Broadway
Sonoma, CA 95476
(707) 935-3377

Summit Bicycles
1820 Fourth Street
San Rafael, CA 94901
(415) 456-4700
www.summitbicycles.com

3 Ring Cycles
1925 Francisco Boulevard East # 18
San Rafael, CA 94901
(415) 259-5704
www.3ringcycles.com

Village Peddler Bicycle Shop
1161 Magnolia Avenue
Larkspur, CA 94939
(415) 461-3091
villagepeddler.com

East Bay

Alamo Bicycles
1483 Danville Boulevard
Alamo, CA 94507
(925) 837-8444

Authorized Bicycle Shop
1220 Georgia Street
Vallejo, CA 94590
(707) 648-1413
www.authorizedbicycle.com

The Bicycle Garage
4673 Thornton Avenue # A
Fremont, CA 94536
(510) 795-9622
www.bicyclegarage.com

Bicycle Outlet
2954 Treat Boulevard
Concord, CA 94518
(925) 687-5970

California Pedaler
495 Hartz Avenue
Danville, CA 94526
(925) 820-0345
www.calped.com

Cyclepath Pleasanton
337B Main Street
Pleasanton, CA 94566
(925) 485-3218
www.cyclepath.com

Danville Bike
115 Hartz Avenue
Danville, CA 94526
(925) 837-0966
www.danvillebike.net

Dublin Cyclery
7001 Dublin Boulevard
Dublin, CA 94568
(925) 828-8676
www.dublincyclery.com

Eden Bicycles
3318 Village Drive
Castro Valley, CA 94546
(510) 881-5000
www.edenbicycles.com

Encina Bicycle Center
2901 Ygnacio Valley Road
Walnut Creek, CA 94598
(925) 944-9200

Fremont Schwinn
4040 Papazian Way
Fremont, CA 94538
(510) 656-8610

Hank & Frank Bicycles
3377 Mount Diablo Boulevard
Lafayette, CA 94549
(925) 283-2453
www.hankandfrankbicycles.com

Jitensha Studio
2250 Bancroft Way
Berkeley, CA 94704
(510) 540-6240
www.jitensha.com

Karim Cyclery
2800 Telegraph Avenue
Berkeley, CA 94705
(510) 841-2181
www.teamkarim.com

Left Coast Cyclery
2928 Domingo Avenue
Berkeley, CA 94705
(510) 204-8550
www.leftcoastcyclery.com

Livermore Cyclery
2752 1st Street
Livermore, CA 94550
(925) 455-8090
www.livermorecyclery.com

Livermore Cyclery: Dublin
7214 San Ramon Road
Dublin, CA 94568
(925) 829-4310
www.livermorecyclery.com

Mike's Bikes of Berkeley
2133 University Avenue
Berkeley, CA 94704
(510) 549-8350
www.mikesbikes.com

Mike's Bikes of Pleasant Hill
1150 Contra Costa Boulevard
Pleasant Hill, CA 94523
(925) 671-9127
www.mikesbicycles.com

Missing Link Bicycle Cooperative
1988 Shattuck Avenue
Berkeley, CA 94704
(510) 843-7471
www.missinglink.org

Pedaler Bike Shop
3826 San Pablo Dam Road
El Sobrante, CA 94590
(510) 222-3420

Pegasus Cycle Works
439 Railroad Avenue
Danville, CA 94526
(925) 362-2220
www.pegasusbicycleworks.com

Perfections Cyclery
2301 Heritage Oaks Drive
Alamo, CA 94507
(925) 260-4647

Performance Bicycle Shop
39121 Fremont Boulevard
Fremont, CA 94538
(510) 494-1466
www.performancebike.com

Performance Bicycle of Walnut Creek
1401 North Broadway
Walnut Creek, CA 94596
(925) 937-7723
www.performancebike.com

Pleasant Hill Cyclery
1100 Contra Costa Boulevard
Pleasant Hill, CA 94523
(925) 676-2667
www.pleasanthillcyclery.com

Pleasanton Bicycles
537 Main Street
Pleasanton, CA 94566
(925) 248-2453
www.bicyclespleasanton.com

REI — Recreational Equipment, Inc.
1338 San Pablo Avenue
Berkeley, CA 94702-1094
(510) 527-4140
www.rei.com

REI — Recreational Equipment, Inc.
1975 Diamond Boulevard
Concord, CA 94520
(925) 825-9400
www.rei.com

Rockville Bike
2635 Springs Road
Vallejo, CA 94591
(707) 648-2453

Sharp Bicycle
969 Moraga Road
Lafayette, CA 94549
(925) 284-9616
www.sharpbicycle.com

Solano Avenue Cyclery
1554 Solano Avenue
Albany, CA 94707
(510) 524-1094
www.solanoavenuecyclery.com

Sports 4 All: Concord
3509 Clayton Road
Concord, CA 94519
(925) 671-9808

Velo-Sport Bicycles
1615 University Avenue
Berkeley, CA 94703
(510) 849-0497
www.velosportbicycles.com

Wheelgirl Bike Shop
1717 Fourth Street, Store C
Berkeley, CA 94710
(510) 524-1400
www.wheelgirl.com

Wrench Science
1022 Murray Street
Berkeley, CA 94710
(510) 841-4748
www.wrenchscience.com

South Bay

Bicycle Express
131 East William Street
San Jose, CA 95112
(408) 998-1618
www.bicycleexpress.net

Bicycle Outfitter
963 Fremont Avenue
Los Altos, CA 94024
(650) 948-8092
www.bicycleoutfitter.com

Bike Connection
2011 El Camino Real
Palo Alto, CA 94306-1124
(650) 853-3000
www.bikeconnection.net

Blastenhoff Custom Bicycle Repair
40 Eureka Square
Pacifica, CA 94044
(650) 359-2700

Calabazas Cyclery
6140 Bollinger Road
San Jose, CA 95129
(408) 366-2453
www.calabazas.com

California Sports & Cyclery
1464 El Camino Real
Belmont, CA 94002
(650) 593-8806
www.californiasportsandcyclery.com

Calmar Bicycles
2236 El Camino Real
Santa Clara, CA 95050
(408) 249-6907
www.calmarcycles.com

Cardinal Bike Shop
1955 El Camino Real
Palo Alto, CA 94306
(650) 328-8900

Chain Reaction Bicycles
1451 El Camino Real
Redwood City, CA 94063
(650) 366-7130
www.chainreactionbicycles.com

Cyclepath of San Mateo
1212 South El Camino Real
San Mateo, CA 94402
(650) 341-0922
www.cyclepath.com

El Camino Bicycle Shop
2320 West El Camino Real
Mountain View, CA 94040
(650) 968-2974
www.offrampbikes.com

Evolution Bike Shop
19685 Stevens Creek Boulevard
Cupertino, CA 95014
(408) 252-5202
www.evolutionbikeshop.com

Fast Bicycle
2274 Alum Rock Avenue
San Jose, CA 95116
(408) 251-9110
www.fastbicycleshop.com

Garners Pro Bike Shop
2755 El Camino Real
Redwood City, CA 94061
(650) 366-2619

Gear Head Bicycles
1039 Terra Nova Boulevard
Pacifica, CA 94044
(650) 359-7185
www.gearheadbikeshop.com

Go Ride Bicycles
2755 El Camino Real
Redwood City, CA 94061
(650) 366-2453
www.goridebicycles.com

Menlo Velo Bicycles
433 El Camino Real
Menlo Park, CA 94025
(650) 327-5137
www.menlovelobicycles.com

Mike's Bikes of Palo Alto
3001 El Camino Real
Palo Alto, CA 94306
(650) 858-7700
www.mikesbikes.com

Palo Alto Bicycles
171 University Avenue
Palo Alto, CA 94301
(650) 328-7411
www.paloaltobicycles.com

Palo Alto Bike Station
95 University Avenue
Palo Alto, CA 94301
(650) 327-9636
www.paloaltobicycles.com

Passion Trail Bikes
415-C Old County Road
Belmont, CA 94002
(650) 620-9798
www.passiontrailbikes.com

Performance Bicycle of Mountain View
2124 West El Camino Real
Mountain View, CA 94040
(650) 964-1796
www.performancebike.com

Performance Bicycle Shop of Redwood City
2535 El Camino Real
Redwood City, CA 94061
(650) 365-9094
www.performancebike.com

REI – Recreational Equipment, Inc.
2450 Charleston Road
Mountain View, CA 94043
(650) 969-1938
www.rei.com

REI – Recreational Equipment, Inc.
1119 Industrial Road
San Carlos, CA 94070
(650) 508-2330
www.rei.com

REI – Recreational Equipment, Inc.
400 El Paseo de Saratoga
San Jose, CA 95130
(408) 871-8765
www.rei.com

Shaw's Lightweight Cycles
45 Washington Street
Santa Clara, CA 95050
(408) 246-7881
www.shawscycles.com

Slough's Bike Shoppe
260 Race Street
San Jose, CA 95126
(408) 293-1616

Specialty Bike Shop
2632 Marine Way
Mountain View, CA 94043
(650) 944-3059

Stanford University: Campus Bike Shop
459 Lagunita Drive
Stanford, CA 94305
(650) 723-9300
www.campusbikeshop.com

Summit Bicycles
1031 California Drive
Burlingame, CA 94010
(650) 343-8483
www.summitbicycles.com

Talbots Cyclery
445 South B Street
San Mateo, CA 94401
(650) 931-8120
www.talbotscyclery.com

Woodside Bike Shop
1523 Woodside Road
Redwood City, CA 94061
(650) 299-1071
www.woodsidebikeshop.com

INDEX

A

Abrigo Valley Trail, 32–33
Alder Spring Trail, 199–200
Almaden Quicksilver County Park, 211–215
Alpine Lake, 91, 94
Alpine Road, 193, 195
animal and plant hazards, 8–10, 181
Annadel State Park
  Canyon Trail and Rough Go Loop, 126–130
  Warren Richardson–North Burma Loop, 131–136
Arastradero Creek, Lake, 183

B

Bass Cove, 28
Bay Area Ridge Trail, 198–199
Bear Creek Staging Area, 29, 31
Berry Creek Ridge, 219, 220
bicycling clubs, 224–225
bicycling retailers, 226–233
Big Basin Redwoods State Park, 216–220
Big D Burgers, 125
Black Diamond Mines Regional Preserve, 59–63
Blue Blossom Trail, 178, 180
Blue Oak Trail, 72–73
Bob Walker Ridge, 71–73
Bobcat Trail, 79–80
Bolinas Beach, Lagoon, 105
Bolinas Ridge Trail, 101–105
Bon Tempe Lake, 91, 94
Boulange de Cole Valley, 153
Briones Regional Park, 29–33
British Bankers Club ("BBC"), restaurant, 190

C

California Coastal Trail project, 83
camping in California, 218
Cañada de Pala Trail, 42– 43
Canyon Trail, 19, 128–129, 140, 203
Capitancillos Ridge, 211
Carbondale Trail, 61–62
Casa Gourmet Burritos, 73
Casa Mexico, 68
Castillero Trail, 213–214
Cave Trail (Trail #20), 120
Cha Cha Cha's, restaurant, 153
Chabot, Anthony, 24, 28
Chausson, Anne-Caroline, 23
China Camp State Park, 96–100
Citrus Club Thai Restaurant, 153
clothing, 5

Clouds Rest Road/Trail, 193, 200
Coal Creek Open Space Preserve, 191–195, 200
Coastal Fire Road, 83–84
Coastal Trail, 78, 80, 83
Cobblestone Trail, 129–130
Contra Loma Regional Park, 62
Creekside Trail, 137, 139
Cybelle's Front Room, restaurant, 148

D

Dalewood Way, 144, 146
de Portola, Gaspar, 156, 160
De Young Museum, 91
Deer Flat, 56, 57
Del Amigo Trail, 34, 38
Devil's Backbone (Trail #25), 120
Diablo Foothills: foothills to Alamo Loop, 44–48
Dipsea Cafe, 85

E

Eagle Loop, Peak, 53, 54
Eagle Springs Backpack Camp, 52
Eagle Trail, 52, 73
East Bay trails, 13–73
East Ridge Trail, 19, 21
East West Cafe, 130
Ed's Mudville Grill, 58
El Corte de Madera Creek Open Space Preserve
  Bear Gulch Loop, 176–180, 190
  Shoots and Ladders, 171–175
El Potrillo Mexican Food, 125
Eldridge Grade, 90–91, 94
El Sombero Taqueria, 18
essentials, 5
Eugene O'Neill National Historic Site, 38

F

Fir Trail, 171, 173, 174
first-aid kit, 7

G

Gazos Creek Road, 218–220
Genghis Khan Kitchen, 28
Chow, restaurant, 33
Golden Gate National Recreation Area, 156
Golden Gate Park (GGP), 91, 151
Gordo's, restaurant, 18
GPS (Global Positioning Satellite)
  See also individual trails
  generally, 1–2

Index

Grabtown Gulch Loop, 166–170
Gravity Car Road, 86, 88
Green Gulch, lookout point, 81
Grizzly Flat, 201, 203, 205
Guadalupe Reservoir, 215

H

Halls Valley Trail, 41, 43
Ha's Restaurant, 38
Hawk Lookout, 79
Helen Putnam Regional Park, 111–115
Hickory Oaks Trail, 208, 210
Highland Ridge Trail, 66–68, 73
Hoo-Koo-E-Koo, 88, 89, 90
Hoover Tower, 200
Hummingbird Trail, 72–73

I

Iron Horse Trail, 36–37

J

Jikoji Zen Center, 206
Jockey Junction (Trail #12), 119
Joseph D. Grant Ranch County Park, 39–43
Juan Bautista de Anza Trail, 183, 185

K

Key at-a-Glance Information, 3
Kezar Bar & Restaurant, 153

L

La Casita Chilanga, 170
Lagunitas Brewery, 93
Lagunitas Rock Springs fire road, 91, 93–94
Lake Camille, 123
Lake Chabot Regional Park, 24–28
Lake Ilsanjo, 128–129, 136
Lake Marie, Road, 123, 124
Lake Trail, 62, 129
Las Trampas Regional Park, 34–38
Laurel Dell fire road, 93
Lawrence Creek Trail, 178, 180
Layang Layang Malaysian Restaurant, 205
Ledson Marsh, 131
Lee's Village Chinese Food, 215
Lepe's Taqueria, 130
Live Oak Trail, 129
Livorna Staging Area, Road, 46, 48
Lo Coco's, 110
Logger's Loop, 27
Lombard Street, 91
Lone Oak picnic area, 16
Lone Ridge Park, 205
Long Ridge Open Space Preserve, 201, 206–210
Los Dos Compadres #2 Taqueria, 220

Los Huercos Trail, 41
Los Vaqueros Reservoir, 73
Lower Lake, 120
Lower Lake Loop (Trail #5), 120
Lower Mystic Trail (Trail #8), 119

M

Madrone Trail, 38
Manzanita Trail, 72–73, 125, 171, 175
maps
    See also specific trails or locations
    directions, 3
    Overview Map and Key, 1
    topo, 5–6
    Trail Maps, 1
Marin Civic Center, 108
Marin Headlands
    Big Southeast Loop with Coastal Trail, 76–80
    Northwest Loop from Tennessee Valley, 81–85
Marincello Trail, 79
Mark West Creek, Trail, 139–140
Marsh Trail, 133–135
Mary's Pizza Shack, 130
Maud Whalen campground, 32
McCarthy, Carl Patrick, 160
McClure Spring, 53
Meadow Trail, 186, 188, 193
Meadowlark Trail, 185
Medical Center Way, 151–152
Menlo Park, 200
Meridian Ridge, Trail, 57–58
Methuselah Trail, 171, 174, 175
Mexican Carniceria, 195
Mextogo, restaurant, 200
Mezue Trail, 17
Mid-peninsula Regional Open Space District, 191, 196
Middle Ridge Road, 219–220
Mill Valley, 86
Mindego Trail, 199
Mine Hill Trail, 211–215
Mini White Moab (MWM), 118–120
Mission Hills Bike Path, 110
Mission Peak, 49–53
Mitchell Canyon Fire Road, 54–58
Miwok, 72, 79–80, 84–85, 99, 111
Monte Bello Open Space Preserve, 201
Monument Peak, 53
Moon Gate, 22
Morgan, Jeremiah, 71
Morgan Territory, 56
Morgan Territory Regional Preserve
    Big Southwest Loop, 64–68
    Volvon Loop Variations, 69–73
Mori Ridge Trail, 156, 158–160

Mott Peak, 29, 32–33
Mount Davidson, 144–149, 153
Mount Diablo, 34, 37, 46–48, 54, 56–57, 62
Mount Diablo State Park, 48, 54–58, 64, 67
Mount Hamilton, 39
Mount Olympia, 58
Mount Sutro, 149–153
Mount Tamalpais State Park
  Hoo-Koo-E-Koo and Old Railroad Grade Loop,
    86–90
  Northern Loop—Rock Spring Road to Eldridge
    Grade via Bon Tempe Lake, 91–95, 109
Mountain Home Inn, 90
Mountain House Restaurant, The, 165
Mountain Mike's Pizza, 215
Mt. Diablo State Park, 44
Murray Park, 89

N

National Mountain Bike Series (NMBS), 57
New Almaden, Trail, 213–214
Nike Missile Site, 159
North Bay trails, 75–141
North Grizzly Flat, 203
North Ridge Trail, 152, 163

O

Oak Ridge Trail, 99
Oakridge Drive Entrance Trail, 119
Ocean View Summit, 219
Oil Canyon Trails, Upper and Lower, 63
Old Adobe Bar & Grill, 125
Old Chicago Pizza, 115
Old Railroad Grade fire road, 88, 90
Old Ranch Road (Trail #23), 119, 120
Olema Inn & Restaurant, 105
Olema Liquor and Deli, 105

P

Pacifica State Beach, 156–160
Pacifica Thai Cuisine, 160
Palo Alto, 181, 185
Panchitos Mexican Restaurant, 110
Panorama Trail, 114–115
Park Chow restaurant, 33
Peak Meadow Trail, 51, 53
Pearson Arastradero Preserve, 181–185
Pelayo's Mexican Restaurant, 120
Peter's Creek Trail, 205, 209–210
Pine Cone Diner, 105
Pizz'a Chicago, 185
Playground, the, 118–119
Point Reyes National Seashore, 104
Pomo Native American Tribe, 111
Pomo Trail, 114–115

Portola Discovery Site, 160
Portola Heights Road, 209
Portola Valley, 186, 189
Potrero Meadow, 93
Providencia Trail, 215
Puerto Alegre Restaurant, 175
Purisima Creek Redwoods
  Grabtown Gulch Loop, 166–170
  Whittemore Wonderland, 161–165

Q

Quarry Trail (Trail #22), 118

R

Railroad Bed Trail, 61
Raleigh's, restaurant, 18
Randall Trail, 105
Randol Trail, 213, 215
Raven Trail, 66, 68
Redwood Bowl Staging Area, 22
Redwood Regional Park, 19–23
Rengstorff Park, 195
Richmond Bridge, 99
Ride Descriptions, 3
Ridge Trail, 113–114, 131, 134, 135, 140
Ridge Trail (The Bay Area Ridge Trail), 205
Ridgewood, 110
Roberts Park Trail, 23
Rock Gardens (Trail #18), 120
Rockville Hills Regional Park, 116–120
Rodeo Lagoon, 78
Rodeo Valley Trail, 79–80
Rough Go Trail, 126, 129–130
Round Valley Regional Park, 73
Russian Ridge Open Space Preserve, 190–191,
  196–200

S

safety, general, 7–8
Salvator Italian Restaurant, 48
San Bruno Mountain, 160
San Francisco area
bicycling clubs, 224–225
bicycling retailers, 226–233
San Francisco Bay, 156, 160
San Francisco Rotary summit garden, 151
San Francisco trails, 143–153
San Jose, 220
San Pablo Ridge, 14, Trail, 18
San Pedro Mountain, 108
Sand Dollar Restaurant, 95
Sandy Point, 220
Santa Isabel Trail, 215
Santa Rosa, 129–130
Sausalito, 79–80, 84

Saylor's South of the Border, 80
Shangri La, restaurant,180
Shell Ridge Open Space, 44, 46
Shiloh Ranch Regional Park, 137–141
Shoreline Trail, 98–99
Shoreline Trailhead, 96
Sierra Azul Open Space Preserve, 211, 214
Sierra Morena Trail, 173
Sindicich Lagoons, 33
Singlespeed World Championships (SSWC) 2008,
    121, 123
Skyline/Buckeye Trails, 123
Skyline Ridge, 163
Skyline Ridge Open Space Preserve, 201, 205
Skyline Wilderness Park: Singlespeeder's Delight,
    121–125
Sleepy Hollow, 106–110
South Bay trails, 155–221
South Skyline Region Open Space Preserve, 196,
    201–205
Spring Board Trail, 176, 179–180
Spring Creek, 128, 130
Spring Ridge Trail, 186, 188, 190
Stevens Creek, 201, 203–204
Stevens Creek Nature Trail, 204–205
Stewartsville Trail, 61–63
Stinson Beach, 95, 105
Stone Corral Trail, 71, 73
Su Casa Mexican Restaurant, 136
Sugarloaf Peak, 124
Sulphur Springs Trail, 67–68
Sweeney Ridge Trail, 156, 158–160

T

Tacos Al Pastor, 215
Tao House, 38
Taqueria El Farolito, 23
Taqueria El Sombrero Numero Dos, 141
Taqueria Salsa, 63
Taqueria San Jose, 43, 100
Tennessee Beach, 81, 83
Tennessee Valley, 76
Tennessee Valley Road, 83
Tennessee Valley Trail, 85
Terra Linda Ridge fire road, 109
Terra Linda/Sleepy Hollow Divide Open Space
    Preserve, 106
Thatchers Rim Rock Trail, 123
Theatre in the Woods, 176
Tia Juana Bar & Grill, 53
Timberview Trail, 171, 175
Tomac, John, 49
Tomales Bay, 103–104
Toyon Canyon Trail, 32–33
Trail #3/Upper Tilly Trail, 120

Trail #5/ Lower Lake Loop, 120
Trail #8/Lower Mystic Trail, 119
Trail #12/Jockey Junction, 119
Trail #14/Unknown Trail, 119
Trail #18/Rock Gardens, 120
Trail #20/Cave Trail, 120
Trail #22/Quarry Trail, 118
Trail #23/Old Ranch Road, 119, 120
Trail #25/Devil's Backbone, 120
trail etiquette, 10
Treasure Island, 99
Two Quarry Trail, 131, 133, 136

U

Unknown Trail (Trail #14), 119
Upper Quarry Trail, 120
Upper Stevens Creek County Park, 201
Upper Steve's Trail, 134
Upper Tilly Trail (Trail #3), 120

V

Valley View Loop, 195
Valley View Trail, 72 –73, 193–194
Volvon Loop Trail, 72–73
Volvon Native American Tribe, 69
Volvon Trail, 71–72

W

Wall, The, 63
Walnut Creek, 46
Warren Richardson Trail, 131, 136
water, 4–5
Water Tower Road, 58
weather, 3–4
West Ridge Trail, 21–22
West Waddell Creek, 220
Whittemore Gulch, 124, 161, 163–164
Wildcat Canyon Regional Park: Havey Canyon to
    Belgum Trail Loop, 14–18
Wildcat Creek Trail, 16, 18
Windy Hill Open Space Preserve: Windy Hill
    Out-and-Back, 186–190
Windy Hill Peak, 190
Wood Trail, 214
World Cup Mountain Bike Races, 121

DEAR CUSTOMERS AND FRIENDS,

SUPPORTING YOUR INTEREST IN OUTDOOR ADVENTURE, travel, and an active lifestyle is central to our operations, from the authors we choose to the locations we detail to the way we design our books. Menasha Ridge Press was incorporated in 1982 by a group of veteran outdoorsmen and professional outfitters. For 25 years now, we've specialized in creating books that benefit the outdoors enthusiast.

Almost immediately, Menasha Ridge Press earned a reputation for revolutionizing outdoors- and travel-guidebook publishing. For such activities as canoeing, kayaking, hiking, backpacking, and mountain biking, we established new standards of quality that transformed the whole genre, resulting in outdoor-recreation guides of great sophistication and solid content. Menasha Ridge continues to be outdoor publishing's greatest innovator.

The folks at Menasha Ridge Press are as at home on a white-water river or mountain trail as they are editing a manuscript. The books we build for you are the best they can be, because we're responding to your needs. Plus, we use and depend on them ourselves.

We look forward to seeing you on the river or the trail. If you'd like to contact us directly, join in at www.trekalong.com or visit us at www.menasharidge.com. We thank you for your interest in our books and the natural world around us all.

SAFE TRAVELS,

Bob Sehlinger

BOB SEHLINGER
PUBLISHER